William H. Clarke

**Horses' Teeth**

a treatise on their mode of development, anatomy, microscopy, pathology, and dentistry, compared with the teeth of many other land and marine animals, both living and extinct

William H. Clarke

**Horses' Teeth**

*a treatise on their mode of development, anatomy, microscopy, pathology, and dentistry, compared with the teeth of many other land and marine animals, both living and extinct*

ISBN/EAN: 9783337235598

Printed in Europe, USA, Canada, Australia, Japan

Cover: Foto ©Andreas Hilbeck / pixelio.de

More available books at **www.hansebooks.com**

A TREATISE ON THEIR

MODE OF DEVELOPMENT, ANATOMY,
MICROSCOPY, PATHOLOGY, AND DENTISTRY; COMPARED WITH
THE TEETH OF MANY OTHER LAND AND MARINE
ANIMALS, BOTH LIVING AND EXTINCT;
WITH A VOCABULARY AND COPI-
OUS EXTRACTS FROM
THE WORKS OF

# ODONTOLOGISTS AND VETERINARIANS.

BY

WILLIAM H. CLARKE.

SECOND EDITION, REVISED.

---

Horses have very nearly the same diseases as men.—*Pliny.*
We ought to make not merely books, but valuable collections, and to acknowledge the sources whence we derive assistance.—*Ibid.*

---

NEW YORK:
WILLIAM R. JENKINS,
VETERINARY PUBLISHER AND BOOKSELLER,
850 SIXTH AVENUE.
1884.

*Copyright, 1879, by* WILLIAM H. CLARKE.

SMITH & McDOUGAL, ELECTROTYPERS,
82 Beekman St., N. Y.

# PREFACE.

THE favorable reception of the first edition of this work by both press and public and my desire to encourage the study of Veterinary Science and Comparative Anatomy are the chief reasons for a Revised Edition. The improvements consist in an Appendix, numerous Illustrations, a new Index, and the correction of errors in and the addition of fresh matter to the text and vocabulary.

I am indebted to Mr. Jacob L. Wortman of Philadelphia for the able article on fossil horses in the Appendix, and to Prof. E. D. Cope, editor of *The American Naturalist*, for a careful revision and improvement of it. Some of the reference notes, however, are my own.

It was not my intention originally to make the book an exponent of the Doctrine of Evolution. The discussion of the subject, however, is justifiable, for a work that does not embrace all the facts science furnishes is unworthy of the age, and to shirk the responsibility of the discussion because the subject is unpopular is cowardly. The fact that fossil horses' teeth are inseparably connected with those of the modern horse renders their consideration unavoidable. Further, in addition to being one of the most important factors Paleontology has thus far furnished in elucidating the subject of Evolution, they give increased scope and importance to the book itself. Truly the late Dr. John W. Draper was right when, at a mere glance, he said: "The subject (horses' teeth) is so suggestive!"

So far as Evolution is concerned, I can only repeat what I said in the first Preface, namely, that it denotes improvement, and that Nature's laws are immutable, and to oppose them is as foolish as to beat the head against a stone wall.

Again, as said in the first Preface, I think I can say now from experience that Special Works, on account of the thoroughness with which they are usually prepared, are growing in public favor (an opinion in which so able a journal as *The Syracuse* (N. Y.) *Standard* concurs), and that while General Works have their advantages, thoroughness of detail is not usually among them.

W. H. C.

NEW YORK, September, 1883.

# CONTENTS.

INTRODUCTION.—Fundamental Principles of Dental Science........ 7

## CHAPTER I.
### TOOTH-GERMS (ODONTOGENY).
Periods at which the Germs are visible in the Fetus.—Dentine and Enamel Germs.—A Cement Germ in the Foal.—The Horse's Upper Grinders said to be developed from Five Germs, the Lower from Four.—Similar development of the Human Teeth.—Monsieur Magitot's Researches.................................................................. 31

## CHAPTER II.
### THE TEMPORARY DENTITION.
Twelve Incisors and Twelve Molars.—Why the Incisors are calle "Nippers."—The Treatment of Foals Affects Teething.—Roots of Milk Teeth Absorbed by the Permanent.—The Tushes.......... 47

## CHAPTER III.
### THE PERMANENT DENTITION.
Distinction between Premolars and Molars.—The Bow-like Incisors.—Contrasts between the Upper and Lower Grinders, and the Rows formed by them.—The Incisors saved from Friction.—Horses' Teeth compared with those of other Animals.—Measurements.—Time's Changes.—Growth during Life............................ 53

## CHAPTER IV.
### THE CANINE TEETH OR TUSHES.
Practically Useless.—Different in their Nature from the other Teeth.—Were they formerly Weapons of Offense and Defense?—Views of Messrs. Darwin, Hunter, Bell, Youatt, and Winter.—Their time of Cutting the most Critical Period of the Horse's Life............... 75

## CHAPTER V.
### THE REMNANT TEETH.
Usually regarded as Phenomenons.—The Name.—Traced to the Fossil Horses, in which (in the Pliocene Period) they "Ceased to be Functionally Developed."—Nature's Metamorphoses.—"The Agencies which are at work in Modeling Animal and Vegetable Forms."—Why Remnant Teeth are often, as it were, Prematurely Lost.—Fossil Horses and a Fossil Toothed-Bird........................... 94

## CHAPTER VI.
### DENTAL CYSTS AND SUPERNUMERARY TEETH.

Teeth growing in various parts of the Body.—Some Cysts more Prolific than others, Producing a Second, if not a Third, "Dentition."—Reports and Theories of Scientific Men.—Cases of Third Dentition in Human Beings. .................................................. 115

## CHAPTER VII.
### HORSES' TEETH UNDER THE MICROSCOPE.

The Dentinal Tubes, Enamel Fibers, and Cemental Canals Described and Contrasted .................................................. 130

## CHAPTER VIII.
### THE PATHOLOGY OF THE TEETH.

Importance of the Subject.—Caries caused by Inflamed Pulps, Blows, Virus, and Morbid Diathesis.—Supernumerary Teeth and other Derangements.—Trephining the Sinuses.—Gutta Percha as a Filling.—Cleaning the Teeth.—A Diseased Fossil Tooth .................. 136

## CHAPTER IX.
### THE DENTISTRY OF THE TEETH.

Reports of Cases Treated by Various Surgeons.—Gutta Percha as a Filling for Trephined Sinuses.—Teeth Pressing against the Palate.—Passing a Probe through a Decayed Tooth.—Death of a Horse from Swallowing a Diseased Tooth .................................. 175

## CHAPTER X.
### FRACTURED JAWS.

How Caused, and how to Distinguish an Abrasion of the Gums from a Fracture of the Bone.—Replacing an Eye, Amputating part of a Lower Jaw, taking a Fractured Tooth and Bones out through the Nostril, &c .................................................. 194

## CHAPTER XI.
### THE TEETH AS INDICATORS OF AGE.

Their various ways of Indicating Age.—The "Mark's" Twofold Use.—The Dentinal Star.—Marks with too much Cement.—Tricks of the Trade.—Crib-biting.—Signs of Age Independent of the Teeth ...... 203

## CHAPTER XII.
### THE TRIGEMINUS OR FIFTH PAIR OF NERVES.

Its Nature and the Relation it bears to the Teeth.—Its Course in the Horse and in Man ............................................. 216

VOCABULARY .................................................. 227

APPENDIX.—Recent Discoveries of Fossil Horses.—Views of an Evolutionist.—Original Home of the Horse.—Elephant Tooth-Germs.—Filling Children's Teeth ....................................... 257

INDEX ....................................................... 279

PUBLIC OPINION .............................................. 287

# INTRODUCTION.

THE following matter, which is designed to give at least a synopsis of the fundamental principles of dental science, is compiled from the works of the best known odontologists. It is somewhat heterogeneous in its make-up, and is, moreover, considering that it is an Introduction to a special work, anomalous, being rather an adjunct to than an explanation of the work itself. Its lack of coherency and the few repetitions, the inevitable concomitants of all compilations, are offset by the interest of its historical records and the scope and clearness of its thoughts and deductions. While it does not treat specially of horses' teeth, it is just as applicable to them as to human teeth, or to those of any of the other animals mentioned. It is believed that the student of dental science will find the matter as useful as it is interesting.

In his work entitled "The Anatomy of Vertebrates" (vol. i, pp. 357–8), Prof. Richard Owen says:

"A tooth is a hard body attached to the mouth or beginning of the alimentary canal, partially exposed, when developed. Calcified teeth are peculiar to the vertebrates, and may be defined as bodies primarily, if not permanently, distinct from the skeleton, consisting of a cellular and tubular basis of animal matter, containing earthy particles, a fluid, and a vascular pulp.

"In general, the earth is present in such quantity as to render the tooth harder than bone, in which case the animal basis is gelatinous, as in other hard parts where a great proportion of earth is combined with animal matter. In a very few instances, among the vertebrate animals, the hardening material exists in a much smaller proportion, and the animal basis is albuminous; the teeth here agree, in both chemical and physical qualities, with bone.

"I propose to call the substance which forms the main part of all teeth dentine.* The second tissue, which is the most exterior in situation, is the cement. The third tissue, which, when present, is situated between the dentine and cement, is the enamel.

"Dentine consists of an organized animal basis and of earthy particles. The basis is disposed in the form

---

* In a reference note in the Introduction to his "Odontography," Prof. Owen says: "Besides the advantage of a substantive for an unquestionably distinct tissue under all its modifications in the animal kingdom, the term dentine may be inflected adjectively, and the properties of this tissue described without the necessity of periphrasis. Thus we may speak of the 'dentinal' pulp, 'dentinal' tubes or cells, as distinct from the corresponding properties of the other constituents of a tooth. The term 'dental' will retain its ordinary sense, as relating to the entire tooth or system of teeth."

*Note.*—The particular paragraph to which the above note refers is from Prof. Owen's "Odontography." "The Anatomy of Vertebrates" having been written about twenty-five years subsequent to the "Odontography," and therefore reflecting the Professor's riper thoughts, the extracts made from it were substituted for very similar matter in the "Odontography."

of compartments or cells, and extremely minute tubes. The earthy particles have a twofold arrangement, being either blended with the animal matter of the interspaces and parietes of the tubes, or contained in a minute granular state in their cavities. The density of the dentine arises principally from the proportion of earth in the first of these states of combination. The tubes contain, near the formative pulp, filamentary processes of that part, and convey a colorless fluid, probably transuded 'plasma.' They thus relate not only to the mechanical conditions of the tooth, but to the vitality and nutrition of the dentine. This tissue has few or no canals large enough to admit capillary vessels with the red particles of blood, and it has been therefore called 'unvascular dentine.'

"Cement always closely corresponds in texture with the osseous tissue of the same animal; and whenever it occurs of different thickness, as upon the teeth of the horse, sloth, or ruminant, it is also traversed, like bone, by vascular canals. When the osseous tissue is excavated, as in dentigerous vertebrates above fishes, by minute radiated cells, forming, with their contents, the 'corpuscles of Purkinjé,' these are likewise present, of similar size and form, in the cement, and are its chief characteristic as a constituent of the tooth. The hardening material of the cement is partly segregated and combined with the parietes of the radiated cells and canals, and is partly contained in disgregated granules in the cells, which are thus rendered white and opaque, viewed by reflected light. The relative density of the dentine and cement varies according to the proportion of the earthy material, and chiefly of that part which is combined with the animal matter in the walls of the cavities, as compared with the size and number of the cavities themselves. In the complex grinders of the elephant, the masked boar, and the copybara, the cement, which forms nearly half the mass of the tooth, wears down sooner than the dentine.

"The enamel is the hardest constituent of a tooth, and, consequently, the hardest of animal tissues; but it consists, like the other dental substances, of earthy matter arranged by organic forces in an animal matrix. Here, however, the earth is mainly contained in the canals of the animal membrane, and, in mammals and reptiles, completely fills those canals, which are comparatively wide, whilst their parietes are of extreme tenuity. The hardening salts of the enamel are not only present in far greater proportion than in the dentine and cement, but, in some animals, are peculiarly distinguished by the presence of the fluate of lime."

Again Prof. Owen says ("Anat. of Vert." vol. i, pp. 359–60):

"Teeth vary in number, size, form, structure, modifications of tissue, position, and mode of attachment in different animals. They are principally adapted for seizing, tearing, dividing, pounding, or grinding the food. In some animals they are modified to serve as weapons of offense and defense; in others, as aids in locomotion, means of anchorage, instruments for uprooting or cutting down trees, or for transport and working of building materials. They are characteristic of age and sex, and in man they have secondary relations subservient to beauty and to speech.

"Teeth are always most intimately related to the food and habits of the animal, and are therefore highly interesting to the physiologist. They form for the same reason most important guides for the naturalist in the classification of animals; and their value, as zoölogical characters, is enhanced by the facility with which, from their position, they can be examined in living or recent animals. The durability of their tissues renders them not less available to the paleontologist in the determination of the nature and affinities of extinct species, of whose organization they are often the sole remains discoverable in the deposits of former periods of the earth's history."

Prof. A. Chauveau says ("Comparative Anatomy of the Domesticated Animals"):

"Identical in all our domesticated animals by their general disposition, mode of development, and structure, in their external conformation the teeth present notable differences, the study of which offers the greatest interest to the naturalist. For it is on the form of its teeth that an animal depends for its mode of alimentation; it is the régime, in its turn, which dominates the instincts, and commands the diverse modifications in the apparatus of the economy; and there results from this law of harmony so striking a correlation between the arrangement of the teeth and the conformation of the other organs, that an anatomist may truly say, 'Give me the tooth of an animal, and I will tell you its habits and structure.'"

In a letter which I wrote to Prof. Theodore Gill, of the Smithsonian Institution. Washington, D. C., I asked what there was about teeth that enabled naturalists to tell so much by them. In reply he said:

"The teeth are quite constant in the same type, are generally appreciably modified according to family, are the most readily preserved in a fossil state, and are in direct relation with the economy of the animal. Hence they furnish the best indications of the relations of the animal to which they belonged, especially in cases where the type was not very different from an existing one. In the case of the older and more aberrant types, however, the indications furnished by the dentition should be accepted with great caution."

In the Introduction to his "Odontography" Prof. Owen gives, besides his own and other men's views, a history "of the leading steps to the present knowledge" of dental science (that is, up to 1844), of which the following are extracts:

"As regards the teeth, the principle of chief import to the physiologist arises out of the fact, which has been established by microscopic investigations, that the earthy particles of dentine are not confusedly blended with the animal basis, and the substance arranged in superimposed layers, but that these particles are built up with the animal basis as a cement, in the form of tubes or hollow columns, in the predetermined arrangement of which there may be discerned the same relation to the acquisition of strength and power of resistance in the due direction, as in the disposition of the columns and beams of a work of human architecture.

"Whoever attentively observes a polished section or a fractured surface of a human tooth may learn, even with the naked eye, that the silky and iridescent luster reflected from it in certain directions is due to the presence of a fine fibrous structure.

"Malpighi,* in whose works may be detected the germs of many important anatomical truths that have subsequently been matured and established, says the teeth consist of two parts, of which the internal bony layers (dentine) seem to be composed of fibrous and, as it were, tendinous capillaments reticularly interwoven.

"Leeuwenhoek,† having applied his microscopical observations to the structure of the teeth, discovered that the apparent fibers were really tubes, and he communicated a brief but succinct account of his discovery to the Royal Society of London, which was published, together with a figure of the tubes, in No. 140 of their *Transactions*. This figure of the dentinal tubes, with additional observations, again appeared in the Latin edition of Leeuwenhoek's works, published at Leyden in 1730. The dentine of the human teeth, and also that of young hogs, is described as being 'formed of tubuli spreading from the cavity in the center to the circumference.' He computed that he saw a hundred and twenty of the tubuli within the forty-fifth part of an inch. He was aware also of the peculiar substance now termed the cement, or *crusta petrosa*, which enters into the composition of the teeth of the horse and the ox.

"These discoveries may be said to have appeared before their time. The contemporaries of Leeuwen-

---

\* An Italian physician; born in 1628; died in 1694. He was the first to apply the newly-invented microscope in the study of anatomy.

† A Dutch naturalist and manufacturer of optical instruments. His microscopes were said to be the best in Europe. Besides his dental discoveries, he discovered the red globules of the blood, the infusorial anima'cules, and that of the spermatozoa. Born in Delft October 24, 1632; died there August 26, 1723.

hock were not prepared to appreciate them; besides they could neither repeat nor confirm them, for his means of observation were peculiarly his own; and hence it has happened that, with the exception of the learned Portal,* they have either escaped notice, or have been designedly rejected by all anatomists until the time of the confirmation of their exactness and truth by Purkinjé in 1835."

Continuing the subject, Prof. Owen further says of the three constituent parts of teeth—dentine, enamel, and cement—beginning with

### THE DENTINE.

"Purkinjé states that the dentine consists, not of superimposed layers, but of fibers arranged in a homogeneous intermediate tissue, parallel with one another, and perpendicular to the surface of the tooth, running in a somewhat wavy course from the internal to the external surface, and he believed these fibers to be really tubular, because on bringing ink into contact with them, it was drawn in as if by capillary attraction.

"On the publication of this discovery, it was immediately put to the test by Prof. Müller, by whom the tubular structure of the dentine was not only confirmed, but the nature and one of the offices of the tubes were determined. He observed that the white color of a tooth was confined to these tubes, which were imbedded in a semitransparent substance, and he found that the whiteness and opacity of the tubes were removed by acids. On breaking a thin lamella of a tooth transversely with regard to its fibers, and examining the edge of the fracture, Müller perceived tubes pro-

---

* "Histoire de l'Anatomie et de la Chirurgie," Paris, 1770.

jecting here and there from the surfaces. They were white and opaque, stiff, straight, and apparently not flexible. This appearance is well represented in the old figure by Leeuwenhoek. If the lamellæ had been previously acted upon by acid, the projecting tubes were flexible and transparent, and often very long. Hence Müller inferred that the tubes have distinct walls, consisting of an animal tissue, and that, besides containing earthy matter in their interior, their tissue is, in the natural state, impregnated with calcareous salts."\*

## THE CEMENT.

"The organized structure and microscopic character of the cement were first determined by Purkinjé and Faenkel, and the acquisition of these facts led to the detection of the tissue in the simple teeth of man and carnivorous animals. The cement is most conspicuous where it invests the root of the tooth, and increases in thickness as it approaches the apex of the root. The animal constituent of this part of the cement had been recognized by Berzelius as a distinct investment of the dentine long before the tissue of which it formed the basis was clearly recognized in simple teeth. Berzelius describes the cemental membrane as being less consistent than the animal basis of the dentine, but resisting

---

\* If Lord Bacon's theory is correct, the probability is that these tubes contain something besides earthy matter and calcareous salts, to wit, *spirit*. In "Novum Organum" he says (B. Montagu, vol. xiv, p. 417): "All things abhor a solution of their continuity, but yet in proportion to their rarity. The more rare the bodies be, the more they suffer themselves to be thrust into small and narrow passages; for water will go into a passage which dust will not go into, air which water will not go into, and flame and spirit which air will not go into."

longer the solvent action of boiling water, and retaining some fine particles of the earthy phosphates when all such earth had been extracted from the dentinal tissue. Cuvier also states that the cement is dissolved with more difficulty in acid than the other dental tissues. Retzius,* however, states that the earth is sooner extracted by acid from the cement than from the dentine of the teeth of the horse.

"In recent mammalian cement the radiated cells, like the dentinal tubes, owe their whiteness and opacity to the earth which they contain. According to Retzius, 'numerous tubes radiate from the cells, which, being dilated at their point of beginning, give the cells the appearance of an irregular star. These tubes form numerous combinations with each other, partly direct and partly by means of fine branches of $\frac{1}{10000}$th to $\frac{1}{50000}$th of an inch in diameter. The cells vary in size. The average size of the Purkinjean cells in human cement is $\frac{1}{1600}$th of an inch. In sections made transversely to the axis of the tooth, it is clearly seen that these cells are arranged in parallel or concentric striæ, of which some are more clearly and others more faintly visible, as if the cement were deposited in fine and coherent layers.' The layer of cement is found in

---

* Prof. Retzius, of the University of Stockholm, informs us that he had been led by the iridescence of the fractured surface of the substance of a tooth to conceive that that appearance was due, as in the crystalline lens, to a fine fibrous structure, and that he communicated his opinions as to the regular arrangement of these fibers to some of his colleagues in 1834. In 1835, having obtained a powerful microscope, he began a series of more exact researches on the intimate structure of the teeth in man and the lower animals, which he communicated to the Royal Academy of Sciences at Stockholm on January 13, 1836, being then unacquainted with the discoveries of Purkinjé.—*Owen.*

the deciduous teeth, but is relatively thinner, and the Purkinjean cells are more irregular.

"'In growing teeth, with roots not fully formed, the cement is so thin that the Purkinjean cells are not visible. It looks like a fine membrane, and has been described as the periosteum of the roots, which are wholly composed of it; but it increases in thickness with the age of the tooth, and is the seat and origin of what are called *exostoses* of the roots.' These growths are subject to the formation of abscesses, and all the morbid actions of true bone.

"It is the presence of this osseous substance which renders intelligible many well-known experiments of which human teeth have been the subjects, such as their transplantation and adhesion into the combs of cocks, and the establishment of a vascular connection between the tooth and the comb.

"Under every modification the cement is the most highly organized and most vascular of the dental tissues, and its chief use is to form the bond of vital union between the denser and commonly unvascular constituents of the tooth and the bone in which the tooth is implanted. In a few reptiles (now extinct), and in the herbivorous mammalia, the cement not only invests the exterior of the teeth, but penetrates their substance in vertical folds, varying in number, form, extent, thickness, and degree of complexity, and contributing to maintain that inequality of the grinding surface of the tooth which is essential to its function as an instrument for the comminution of vegetable substances."\*

---

\* CEMENT MISTAKEN FOR TARTAR (ODONTOL'ITHOS).—Surgeon E. Mayhew says ("The Horse's Mouth," &c.): "Within the alveolar cavity, the crusta petrosa, which becomes of con-

## THE ENAMEL.

"The higher an animal is placed in the scale of organization, the more distinct and characteristic are not only the various organs of the body, but the different tissues which enter into their composition. This law is well exemplified in the teeth, although in the comparison of these organs we are necessarily limited to the range of a single primary group of animals. We have seen, for example, that the dentine is scarcely distinguishable from the tissue of the skeleton in the majority of fishes; but that its peculiarly dense, unvascular, and resisting structure, which is the exceptionable condition in fishes, is its prevalent character in the teeth of the higher vertebrates.

"So likewise with the enamel. This substance, which under all its conditions bears a close analogy with the dentine, is hardly distinguishable from that tissue in the teeth of many fishes. The fine calcigerous* tubes are present in both substances, and undergo similar subdivisions, the directions only of the trunks

siderable thickness around the root, is of a yellowish-white color; but where, as on the crown of the tooth, it is exposed to the chemical action of food and air, it presents a darker aspect, and resembles an accumulation of tartar, for which indeed it has been mistaken. It fills up the infundibula of the grinders and lines those of the incisors. It is pierced by all the vessels which nourish the teeth."

The editor of "The Veterinarian" (1849), in a "review" of Mr. Mayhew's work, says: "Both English and French veterinary writers have mistaken the crusta petrosa for tartar, not being aware of its existence inside as well as outside of the tooth."

\* This word is peculiar to if not originated by Prof. Owen. It is synonymous with the word *Calciferous* (limy).

and branches being reversed, agreeably with the contrary course of their respective developments. The proportion of animal matter is also greater in the enamel of the teeth of fishes than in the higher vertebrata, and the proportion of the calcareous salts incorporated with the animal constituent of the walls of the tubes is greater as compared with the subcrystalline part deposited in the tubular cavities.

"The enamel may be distinguished, independently of its microscopic and structural characters, by its glistening, subtransparent substance, which is white or bluish-white by reflected light, but of a gray-brown color when viewed, under the microscope, by transmitted light. * * * The enamel of the molar tooth of a calf, which has just begun to appear above the gum, and which can readily be detached from the dentine, especially near the beginning of the roots, is resolvable into apparently fine prismatic fibers. If these fibers be separately treated with dilute muriatic acid, and the residue examined with a moderate magnifying power, in distilled water, or, better, in dilute alcohol, portions of more or less perfect membranous sheaths or tubes will be discerned, which inclosed the earthy matter of the minute prism, and served as the mold in which it was deposited.

"Prof. Retzius, who obtained a small portion of organic or animal substance from the enamel-fibers of an incompletely-formed tooth of a horse, conjectured that it was a deposition of that fluid which originally surrounds the loose enamel-fibers, and that 'in proportion as these fibers are pressed tighter together, and additional fibers are wedged between them, the organic deposition is forced away.'

"Retzius accurately describes the enamel-fibers of

the horse as presenting the form of angular needles, about $\frac{1}{8000}$th of an inch in diameter, which are traversed by minute and close-set transverse striæ over the whole or a part of the fiber; and he conjectures that if the enamel-fiber be a mass of the calcareous salts, surrounded by an organic capsule, that the striæ may then belong to the capsule, and not to the enamel-fiber. The later researches of Dr. Schwann add to the probability of this conjecture; and the absence of the minute striæ in the enamel of fossil mammalian teeth, at least in the examples which I have submitted to microscopic investigation, may depend upon the destruction of the original organic constituent of the enamel.

"The enamel-fibers are directed at nearly right angles to the surface of the dentine, and their central or inner extremities rest in slight but regular depressions on the periphery of the coronal dentine. Thus in the human tooth, the fibers which constitute the masticating surface are perpendicular, or nearly so, to that surface, while those at the lower part of the crown are transverse, and consequently have a position best adapted for resisting the pressure of the contiguous teeth, and for meeting the direction in which external forces are most likely to impinge upon the exposed crown of the tooth. The strength of the enamel-fibers is further increased by the graceful, wavy curves in which they are disposed. These curves are in some places parallel, in others opposed. Their concavities are commonly turned toward each other, where the shorter fibers, which do not reach the exterior of the enamel, abut by their gradually attenuated peripheral extremities upon the longer fibers. Other shorter fibers extend from the outer surface of the enamel toward the dentine, and are wedged into the interspaces of the longer fibers. In the teeth of fishes, the calcigerous tubes or fibers of the enamel, which ramify and subdivide like those of the dentine, have their trunks turned in the opposite direction, or toward the periphery of the tooth. So likewise in human teeth the analogous condition may be discerned in the slightly augmented diameter of the enamel-fibers at their peripheral as compared with their central extremities. When the extremities of the human enamel-fibers are examined with a magnifying power of 300 linear dimensions, by reflected light, they are seen to be co-adapted, like the cells of a honey-comb, and, like these, to be, for the most part, hexagonal.

"The internal surface of the enamel is marked by fine transverse lines or ridges, of which Retzius counted twenty-four in the vertical extent of one-tenth of an English inch of the crown of a human incisor. These lines are parallel and wavy, and, like the analogous markings on the surface of shells, indicate the successive formation of the belts of enamel-fibers that encircle the crown of the tooth. They may be traced around the whole crown, but are very faint upon its inner or posterior surface. Retzius cites Leeuwenhoek as the discoverer of these superficial transverse lines of the enamel, but the older observer supposed them to be indicative of the intervals between the successive movements in the cutting of the tooth through the gum.

"The enamel, by virtue of its physical qualities of density and durability, forms the chief mechanical defense of the tooth, and is consequently limited in most simple teeth to the exterior surface of the exposed portion of the dentine, forming the crown of the tooth. \* \* \* In the herbivorous mammalia, with the exception of the Edentata, vertical folds or processes of the enamel are continued into the substance of the tooth, varying in number, form, extent, and direction, and producing, by their superior density and resistance, the ridged inequalities of the grinding surface on which its efficacy in the trituration of vegetable substances depends."

Dr. Boon Hayes's thoughts are thus recorded in a "Medical Circular," extracts from which appear in "The Veterinarian" for 1853 (pp. 535-6):

"In the first place, observe the pulpal cavity, which is to the tooth what the medullary cavity is to bone. Both originate in the same way. Into it passes an artery, a vein, and a nerve. These ramify upon the pulpal surface, the artery carrying blood to the dentinal tubuli, whence the *liquor sanguinis* (not blood corpuscles) proceeds to the nourishment of this apparently inorganic mass.

"In the teeth of some animals this cavity seems to send off diverticula between the dentinal tubuli, as if for the purpose of supplying them with more vascularity. The dentinal tubes open on the walls of the pulpal cavity, and thence radiate to the enamel superiorly and the crusta petrosa inferiorly. I think it would not be difficult to prove that caries of the teeth more frequently proceeds from inflammation beginning in this cavity than from any other cause.

"When the tubes of the dentine are examined with a high magnifying power, and by transmitted light, they appear dark. They are much more minute in diameter than the blood globules; hence the *liquor sanguinis* alone can penetrate them for their nourishment; so that the teeth are in the same condition as bone in this respect.

"The dentinal tubes, as before said, appear dark; the lighter and apparently broader masses are the real substance of the dentine. In this, and especially near the layer closest to the enamel, dentinal cells are sometimes seen, which may probably be analogous to the lacunæ of bone.

"If the dentinal curvatures are examined, it will be seen that they are of two kinds. One set is in bold and evident curves; the other is not so evident, but it exists, nevertheless, and a little patience and a high magnifying power will demonstrate the fact that its curves are *upon* the curves of the first set. The former are called the primary, the latter the secondary curves of the dentinal tubuli (in botanical description, a biserrated leaf). From the tubuli minute bracelets are given off on the sides, and toward the end the tubes terminate, either in cells, by anastomosis, or by looping back upon themselves.

"The cement at first envelops the whole tooth, but soon wears off the crown and as far down as the neck. Compared with the dentine and enamel, it is very soft, and more closely resembles bone; in fact in some animals it is continuous with the bone of the jaw, thus proving its identity. It contains lacunæ and canaliculi, and, when there is a large mass of it, something like Haversian canals.

"There is a great analogy between tooth and bone. In the cement there is absolute likeness, and in the dentine analogies too striking to be overlooked, viz., the tubuli, analogous to the canaliculi, the intertubular cells, analogous to the lacunæ, and the intertubular substance, analogous to the laminæ of bone. In the enamel the greatest departure is observable, but not wider than its peculiar function suggests; and it must be remembered, first, that it is the least constant tissue of the teeth; secondly, that its chemical composition is very much the same as that of the dentine and cement, both of which resemble bone. Lastly, the analogy is completed in a review of the mode of tooth development. Thus, upon a mucous papilla a large quantity of gelatinous matter is observable, in which certain cells appear. The gelatinous matter resembles the incipient cartilage in which ossification begins. This papilla is supplied with an artery, which nourishes its cells, and the cells gradually so develop that the older ones are pushed outward and form the dentine."

### HOW MADDER AFFECTS THE TEETH.

John Hunter, one of the most celebrated physiologists of the eighteenth century, made many experiments on the teeth of different animals, one object being to determine whether they were vascular or not. His conclusion was that they were not vascular, and he founded his belief partly upon the following experiment ("The Human Teeth," pp. 23-4):

"Take, for example, any young animal, as a pig, and feed it with madder for three or four weeks; then kill it. On examination you will find the following appearances: First, if the animal had some parts of its teeth formed before the feeding with madder, they will be known by their remaining of the natural color; but such parts of the teeth as were formed while the animal was taking the madder will be of a red color. This shows that it is only those parts that were formed while the animal was taking the madder that are dyed;

for what were already formed will not be in the least tinged. This is different in all other bones; for we know that any part of a bone which is already formed is capable of being dyed with madder, though not so fast as the part that is forming. Therefore, as we know that all other bones are vascular, and are thence susceptible of the dye, we may readily suppose that the teeth are not susceptible of it after being once formed. But we shall carry this a step further: If you feed a pig with madder for some time, and then leave it off for a time before killing it, you will find the appearances as above, with this addition, that all the parts of the teeth which were formed after leaving off feeding with the madder will be white. Here, then, in some teeth we shall have white, then red, and then white again; and so we shall have the red and white colors alternately through the whole tooth.*

"This experiment shows that a tooth, once tinged, does not lose its color. Now, as all other bones that

---

* In the concluding part of Moore's "Lalla Rookh" ("The Light of the Harem"), the Enchantress says of an herb with the unmusical name of "Haschischat ed dab:"

"The visions, that oft to worldly eyes
 The glitter of mines unfold,
Inhabit the mountain-herb, that dyes
 The tooth of the fawn like gold."

A reference note to the above is as follows: "An herb on Mount Libanus, which is said to communicate a yellow golden hue to the teeth of the goats and other animals that graze upon it. Niebuhr thinks this may be the herb which the Eastern alchemists look to as a means of making gold. 'Most of those alchemical enthusiasts think themselves sure of success if they could but find out the herb which gilds the teeth and gives a yellow color to the flesh of the sheep that eat it. Even the oil of this plant must be of a golden color. It is called *Haschischat ed dab*.' Father Jerome Dandini, however, asserts that the teeth of the

have been tinged lose their color in time, when the animal leaves off feeding with the madder (though very slowly), and as that dye must be taken into the constitution by the absorbents, it seems that the teeth are without absorbents as well as other vessels."

The editor of Hunter's "Treatise," Thomas Bell, F.R.S., differed with Hunter about the vascularity of the teeth. He thus concludes a note on the above quotation:

"The truth appears to be that the teeth are organized bodies, having nerves and absorbent and circulating vessels, but possessing a low degree of living power, and so dense a structure as to exhibit phenomena, both in their healthy and diseased condition, which are very dissimilar from those which are observed in true osseous structures."

### TRANSPLANTING TEETH.

The transplanting of teeth, which Dr. Hunter says is "similar to the ingrafting of trees," is expatiated upon at some length. He then gives an account of a case of transplanting which he admits "is not generally attended with success," he having "succeeded but once out of a great number of trials." It is as follows ("The Human Teeth," pp. 100–101):

"I took a sound tooth from a person's head; then

goats at Mount Libanus are of a *silver* color, and adds: 'This confirms to me that which I observed in Candia, to wit, that the animals that live on Mount Ida eat a certain herb which renders their teeth of a golden color, which, according to my judgment cannot otherwise proceed than from the mines which are under ground.'—*Dandini, Voyage to Mount Libanus.*"

made a wound in a cock's comb, pressed the root into it, and fastened it with threads. The cock was killed some months after, and I injected the head with a very minute injection. I then put the comb into a weak acid. The tooth was softened, and I divided it longitudinally. Its vessels were well injected, the external surface adhering to the comb by vessels similar to the union of a tooth with the gum and sockets."*

* MM. E. Magitot, C. Legros, and C. Robin have experimented in transplanting the *follicles* or *germs* of dogs' teeth, an account of which appears in "Comptes Rendus" for 1874. They say:

"Our experiments comprised 88 grafts, mostly from newly-born dogs, but some were 22 and even 58 days old. The animals were invariably sacrificed by the pricking of the bulbs, and the jaws were opened at once, to lay the follicles bare. One-half of both jaws thus served to supply the grafts, while the other was kept for a standard of comparison. The dogs on which the grafts were applied were usually adults, but sometimes of the same age and bearing as those that supplied them. The germs were rapidly isolated from the dental gutters, and introduced at once. In some instances they were dipped for a few minutes in the blood's serum of the sacrificed animal, which was kept by the bath (bain-marie) at a temperature of from 30° to 35° C. They were introduced under the skin of the nape of the neck, the top of the head, and the dorsal and lumbar regions. In 36 cases the process of application consisted of a simple incision and the introduction of the graft 2 or 3 centimeters from the opening, which was closed by two sutural stitches. In the other 52 cases a special trocar of an interior diameter of 7 millimeters was used, which allowed a swifter and surer transplantation, but it did not appear to exert an appreciable influence on the results.

"Ten grafts were made from newly-born dogs on adult guinea-pigs, divided as follows: Whole follicles, 6; isolated enamel-organs, 3; bulb alone, 1. The results were all negative—caused by resorption and suppuration—corroborating M. Bert's experiences in grafts between animals of different zoological orders.

"The 78 other grafts were made on newly-born, young, and adult dogs, and were maintained from 13 to 54 days. The 25 grafts that remained 54 days resorbed themselves. The experiments in detail were as follows: 1. Isolated whole follicles, 26. 2. Follicles with a portion of the maxillary bone, 5. 3. Isolated

This appears to prove that Dr. Hunter was right when he said that teeth "are capable of uniting with bulbs, 16. 4. Bulbs with a cap of rudimentary dentine, 7. 5. Isolated caps of dentine, 4. 6. Isolated enamel-organs, with a shred of buccal mucous membrane, 19. 7. Enamel-organs, with a cap of dentine adhering, 1. The results were: Of the first, 7 kept alive and grew steadily, except in one instance, in which a disturbed nutrition brought on the formation of globulary dentine and irregular stacks of enamel prisms. The second gave 3 suppurations and 2 resorptions, again corroborating Mons. Bert's experiments. The third gave 3 positive results, in two of which a new cap of dentine was produced, quite regular, but globulous and somewhat altered in its nutrition. The other was without enamel. In the fourth experiment the bulbs could not be found; they underwent resorption. When compared with the preceding experiment, this result is astonishing; but it should be understood that these grafts were maintained from 43 to 51 days. Of the fifth a single one kept alive, but without showing any growth. It remained stationary 43 days. The sixth invariably ended in resorption, notwithstanding we were careful to graft the shred of mucous membrane, which supplies the organ with nutritive vessels. This result is not surprising when the excessive frailty of this tissue and its lack of vascularity are considered. Some of the negative grafts were either reduced in size, being evidently in process of resorption, or underwent the oily transformation. Others caused abscesses, and were eliminated.

"*Conclusions.*—1. The grafts gave favorable results only between animals of the same zoological order. 2. The isolated whole follicles and bulbs may live and develop themselves. 3. The transplanting of more or less voluminous portions of jaws with the follicles failed through suppuration or resorption. 4. The grafts of the enamel organ, isolated, seem invariably given up to resorption. 5. Under certain circumstances the growth is regular, with no other difference from that in the normal state than a noticeable slowness in the phenomena of evolution. 6. Under other circumstances there is trouble in the formation of the dentine and enamel, the study of which, however, may be applied to the elucidation of the phenomena, still so dark, of tooth development. 7. The experiments are an acquisition to the literature of and may be compared with other surgical grafts."*

---

* For the translation of the above interesting article (from the Reports of the French Academy) I am indebted to Monsieur C. Raoux, of New York.

any part of a living body." Mr. Bell thus concludes a note on the above case of transplanting:

"The experiment has an interest attached to it far more important than its having given rise to the temporary adoption of an objectionable operation. In the result of this experiment may be found an interesting collateral argument in favor of the organized structure of the teeth, and their actual living connection with the body. The vessels of the tooth, we are told, were well injected, and the external surface adhered everywhere to the comb by vessels. To what purpose are these vessels formed, what object can be possibly fulfilled by the existence of a vascular pulp in the internal cavity, and a vascular periosteum covering the external surface—so obviously vascular that it was *well* injected from the vessels of a cock's comb, into which it had been transplanted—unless they are intended to *nourish* the bony substance of which the tooth consists, and to form the medium of its connection with the general system?"

Prof. Richard Owen says ("Odontography," vol. i, p. 470):

"The saving of material is the least of the benefits gained by this tubular structure of the dentine. The vitality of the tissue, which Hunter recognized so forcibly, but which, being equally convinced of the non-vascularity of the tissue, he was unable to explain —'willing rather to enunciate an apparent paradox or be taunted with dilemma, than yield one iota of either of his convictions'*—is explicable by the possible and

* Prof. Owen quotes from Bell's "notes" in Hunter's "Human Teeth."

highly probable fact of a circulation of the colorless plasma of the blood through the dentinal tubes. That some elementary prolongations of nerve may also be continued into these tubes, who can confidently deny?"

As Prof. Owen says the "teeth are always most intimately related to the food and habits of the animal," it would be interesting and perhaps useful to ascertain what effect sugar and other unusual articles of diet would have on horses' teeth. In the interest of science, experiments appear to be in order. In this connection the following paragraph, a part of which may be found in Prof. William Youatt's work, "The Horse" (p. 135), the remainder in "The Veterinarian," is interesting:

"Surgeon Black, of the Fourteenth Dragoons, says that sugar was tried as an article of food during the Peninsular War. Ten horses were selected, each of which got eight pounds a day. They took it very readily, and their coats became fine, smooth, and glossy. They got no corn, and only seven pounds of hay instead of twelve, the ordinary allowance. The sugar supplied the place of corn so well, that it would probably have been given abroad; but peace came, and with it corn. The horses returned to their usual diet, but several of them became crib-biters. The experiment was made at the Brighton dépôt, during a period of three months. To prevent the sugar from being used for other purposes, it was scented with assafetida, but the latter did not produce any apparent effect on the horses."

# HORSES' TEETH.

## CHAPTER I.

### TOOTH-GERMS (ODONTOGENY).

Periods at which the Germs are visible in the Fetus.—Dentine and Enamel Germs.—A Cement Germ in the Foal.—The Horse's Upper Grinders said to be developed from Five Germs, the Lower from Four.—Similar development of the Human Teeth.—Mousieur Magitot's Researches.

FURROWS in what is subsequently transformed into jawbones, in which tooth-germs are, as it were, planted, are Nature's first visible preparation for the development of the teeth. According to Prof. William Youatt, the germs of the temporary teeth are visible seven or eight months before the foal is born. Three months before its birth the germs of the permanent teeth are also visible, a distinct partition separating them from the temporary. At this time, according to Veterinary Dentist C. D. House, the capsules or bags (also called follicles, sacs, &c.), containing the tooth-pulps* of the

---

\* The pulp in the cavity of a *full-grown* tooth is a delicate mass of connective tissue, containing both blood-vessels and nerves. Its external layer consists of large nucleated cells, the odontoblasts, provided with long branching processes which line the dental canals. Boll thinks the nerves' delicate terminal fibrils accompany the processes into the canals.—*Woodward.*

For development of elephant tooth-germs see Appendix.

future temporary teeth are about the size of small peas. They will bear some pressure between the fingers, the indentions springing back like those of an India rubber ball.

The nature of tooth-germs and the development of teeth have been studied with some diligence by scientific men—Dr. John Hunter, it is said, making the first important discoveries in connection with the science. The discussion of this interesting and, to students, useful subject is left to these men. There is some conflict in their views, but it should be remembered that the extracts reflect the opinions of men from Hunter's time (over a century ago), to 1876. The development of tooth-germs being the same in principle (though different in detail) in all mammals, the matter which follows (as has been said of that in the "Introduction"), is as applicable to the horse as to man.

In the Introduction to his "Odontography" (London, 1844), Prof. Richard Owen says:

"In the development of a tooth a matrix of equal complexity was first recognized to be concerned by John Hunter, the several parts of this matrix being first distinctly indicated in the 'Natural History of the Human Teeth.' * * * Hunter has been generally regarded by physiologists as being the author of the theory that the pulp stood to the tooth-bone in the relation of a gland to its secretion; that the formative virtue of the pulp resided in its surface; that the dentine was deposited upon and by the formative or secretive surface in successive layers, and that the pulp, exhausted, as it were, by its secretive activity, diminished in size as the formation of the tooth proceeded, except in certain species, in which it was persistent, and maintained an equable secretion of the dentine throughout the lifetime of the animal. This idea of the pulp's function has predominated in the minds of most subsequent writers on the development of the teeth. \* \* \* \*

"Three formative organs are developed for the three principal or normal dental tissues, the 'dentinal-pulp,' or pulp proper, for the dentine, the 'capsule' for the cement, and the 'enamel-pulp' for the enamel. The essential fundamental structure of each formative organ is cellular, but the cells differ in each organ, and derive their specific characters from the properties and metamorphoses of their nucleus, upon which the specific microscopical characters of the resulting calcified substances depend.

"In the cells of the dentinal-pulp the nucleus fills the parent cell with a progeny of nucleoli before the work of calcification begins. In the enamel-pulp the nucleus of the cell disappears, like the cytoblast of the embryo plant in the formation of most vegetable tissues. In the cells of the capsule the nucleus neither perishes nor propagates, but retains its individuality, and gives origin to the most characteristic feature of the cement, viz., the radiated cells.

"The primordial material of each constituent of the tooth-matrix is derived from the blood, and special arrangements of the blood-vessels preëxist to the development and growth of the constituent substances. A pencil of capillaries is directed to a particular spot in the primitive dentiparous groove, and terminates there by a looped network, from which spot a group of nucleated cells begins to arise in the form of a papilla.

\* \* \* \* \*

"The primary dentinal papilla and its capsule rapidly increase by successive additions of nucleated cells, apparently derived from material supplied by the capillary plexus at the base. The capillaries now begin to penetrate the substance of the pulp itself, where they present a subparallel or slightly diverging pencillate arrangement, but preserve their looped and reticulate termination near the apex of the pulp. Fine branches of nerves accompany the capillaries, and terminate also in loops. * * * The primary cells and the capillary vessels and nerves are imbedded in and supported by a homogeneous, minutely subgranular, mucilaginous substance, the 'blastema.' * * * The vascularity of the dentinal-pulp, and especially the rich network of looped capillaries that adorns the formative peripheral layer at the period of its functional activity, have attracted general notice, and have been described by Hunter and subsequent authors. By most this phenomenon has been regarded as evidence of the secreting function of the surface of the pulp, and the dentine as an outpouring from that vascular surface which was supposed to shrink or withdraw from the matter excreted. * * *

"The enamel-pulp differs from the dentinal-pulp at its first formation by the more fluid state of its blastema, and by the fewer and more minute cells which it contains. The source of this fluid blastema appears to be the free inner vascular surface of the capsule. As it approaches the dentinal-pulp the blastema acquires more consistence by an increased number of its granules, and it contains more numerous and larger cells. Many of these show a nuclear spot, others a nucleus and nucleolus. The spherical nucleolar cells in the part of the blastema further from the capsule are so numerous as to form an aggregate mass, with a small quantity of the condensed blastema in the minute interspaces left between the cells, which are pressed together into hexagonal or polygonal forms. * * * The field of the final metamorphosis of the cells into the molds for the reception of the solidifying salts is confined to close contiguity with the surface of the dentinal-pulp. Here the cells increase in length, lose all trace of their nucleus, and become converted into long and slender cylinders, usually pointed at both ends, and pressed by mutual contact into a prismatic form. These cylinders have the property of imbibing the calcareous salts of the enamel from the plasmatic fluid, and of compacting them in a clear and almost crystalline state in their interior. * * *

"The blastema or fundamental tissue of the capsule is, at first, semitransparent and of a pearly or opaline color, but is soon richly ornamented by the plexiform distribution of the blood-vessels. As the period of its calcification approaches, which is later than that of the dentinal-pulp, it becomes denser, and exhibits numerous nucleated cells. The blastema itself presents more evidently a fine cellular or granular structure, in which the calcareous salts are impacted in a comparatively clear state, constituting the framework of the cemental tissue. The characteristic features of this tissue are due to the action of the proper nucleated cells upon the salts of the plasma diffused through the blastema in which those cells are imbedded, the cells being characterized by a single, large, granular nucleus, which almost fills the clear area of the cell itself. If, when the formation of the cement has begun in the incisor or molar of a colt, one of the detached specks of that substance, with the surrounding and adhering part of the inner surface of the capsule in which it is imbedded, be examined, the nucleated cells are seen, closely aggregated around the calcified part, in concentric rows, the cells of which are further apart as the rows recede from the field of calcification. Those next the cement rest in cup-shaped cavities in the periphery of the calcified part, just as the first calcified cells of the thick cement which covers the crown of a complex molar are lodged in cavities on the exterior of the enamel. These exterior cavities of the cement are formed by centrifugal extension of the calcifying process in the blastema in which the cells are imbedded. The calcareous salts penetrate in a clearer and more compact state the cavity of the cell, but their progress is arrested apparently by the nucleus, which maintains an irregular area, partly occupied by the salts in a subgranular, opake condition, but chiefly concerned in the reception and transit of the plasmatic fluid, which enters and escapes by the minute tubes that are subsequently developed from the nucleolar cavity as calcification proceeds.

"The radiated cells or cavities thus formed are the most common characteristic of the cement, but not the constant one. The layer of the capsule which surrounds the crown of the human teeth and of the simple teeth of quadrumana and carnivora, consists simply of the granular blastema, without nucleated cells, and the radiated corpuscles are, consequently, not developed in the cement which results from its calcification. In the thicker part of the inflected folds of the capsule of the complex teeth of the herbivora, traces of the vascularity of that part of the matrix are persistent, the blastema calcifying around certain of the capillaries, and forming the medullary canals. The varieties of these canals are traversed by minute tubules, continued from or communicating with the radiated cells. These tubules, and the more parallel ones which traverse the thickness of the cement in many mammalia, are the remains of linear series of the minute granules of the blastema.   \*   \*   \*

"The general form of the dental matrix and its relation with its calcified product, bear a close analogy with those of the formative organ of hairs, bristles, and other productions of the epidermal system. In these the papilla, or pulp, is developed from the external skin; in the teeth, from the mucous membrane, or internal skin."   \*   \*   \*   \*

Prof. Charles S. Tomes, among dentists a recognized authority, differs with Messrs. Hunter and Owen as to the pulp's secretive office, claiming that a tooth is formed by a partial metamorphosis of its pulp. He says ("Manual of Dental Anatomy, Human and Comparative," pp. 104-5-6):

"Prior to the beginning of any calcification, there is always a special disposition of the soft tissues at the spot where a tooth is destined to be formed, and the name of 'tooth-germ' is given to those portions of the soft tissue which are thus specially arranged. All, or a part only, of the soft structures making up a tooth-germ become converted into the dental tissue by a deposition of salts of lime within their own substance, so that an actual conversion of at least some portions of the germ into tooth takes place. The tooth is not secreted or excreted by the germ, but an actual metamorphosis of the latter takes place.

"The principal tissues, namely, dentine, enamel, and cement, are formed from different parts of the tooth-germ; hence we are accustomed to speak of the enamel-germ and the dentine-germ. The existence of a special cement-germ is very doubtful, some writers asserting, others denying its existence. \* \* \*

"Tooth-germs are never formed upon the surface, but are situated a little distance beneath it, lying in some animals at a considerable depth. Every known tooth-germ consists in the first instance of two portions, and two only, the enamel and dentine germs. These are derived from distinct sources, the former being a special development from the epithelium of the mouth, the latter from the more deeply lying parts of the mucous membrane. Other things, such as a tooth-capsule, may be subsequently and secondarily formed. The existence of an enamel-organ in an early stage is independent of any subsequent formation of enamel by its own conversion into a calcified tissue, for I have shown it to be found in the germs of teeth which have no enamel; in fact, in all tooth-germs whatever.

"That part of the tooth-germ destined to become dentine is often called the dentine papilla, having acquired this name from its papilliform shape; and in a certain sense it is true that the enamel-organ is the epithelium of the dentine papilla. Yet, although not absolutely untrue, such an expression might mislead by implying that the enamel organ is a secondary development, whereas its appearance is contemporaneous with, if not antecedent to, that of the dentine-germ. The most general account that I am able to give of the process is, that the deeper layer of the oral epithelium sends down into the subjacent tissue a process, the shape and structure of which is, in most animals, distinguishable and characteristic before the dentine-germ has taken any definite form. This process enlarges at its end, and, as seen in section, becomes divaricated, so that it bears some resemblance to an inverted letter Y; or it might be better compared to a bell-jar with a handle. This constitutes the early stage of an enamel-germ, while beneath it, in the mucous tissue, the dentine-germ assumes its papilliform shape. The details of the process varying in different animals, I will at once proceed to the description of the development of teeth in the various groups."

Prof. Tomes's views of the development of tooth-germs in mammals are thus summarized by himself ("Philosophical Transactions Royal Society," 1875, part i, p. 285):

"1. There is never, at any stage, an open groove from the bottom of which papillæ rise up.

"2. That the first recognizable change in the region of a forming tooth-germ is a dipping down of a process of the oral epithelium, looking, in section transverse to the jaw, like a deep simple tubular gland, which descends into the submucous tissue, and ultimately forms the enamel-organ.

"3. That subsequently to the descent of the so-called enamel-germ, the changes in the subjacent tissue resulting in the formation of the dentine papilla take place opposite to its end, and not at its surface.

"4. That the permanent tooth-germs first appear as offshoots from the epithelial process concerned in the formation of the deciduous tooth-germ (Kölliker), the first permanent molar being derived from a primary dipping down (like a deciduous tooth), the second deriving its enamel-germ from the epithelial neck of the first, and the third from that of the second (Legros and Magitot)."

Again, in the Society's *Transactions* for 1876 (p. 265), Prof. Tomes says:

"1. It is desirable to abandon the terms 'papillary,' 'follicular,' and 'eruptive' stages, inasmuch as they are hypothetical and arbitrary, and correspond to no serial conditions verified by observation.

"2. In all animals a tooth-germ consists primarily of two structures, and only two—the dentine-germ and the enamel-germ. The simplest tooth-germ never comprises anything more. When a capsule is developed, it is derived partly from a secondary upgrowth of the tissue at the base of the dentine germ, and partly from an accidental condensation of the surrounding connective tissue.

"3. The existence of an enamel-organ is quite universal, and is in no way dependent on the presence or absence of enamel on the completed tooth, although the degree to which it is developed has distinct relation to the thickness of the future enamel.

"4. So far as my researches go, a stellate reticulum, constituting a large bulk of the enamel-organ, is a structure confined to the mammalia. (It is absent in the armadillo, and I should infer from Mr. Turner's description, in the narwhal also).

"5. As laid down by Profs. Huxley and Kölliker, the dentine-papilla is beyond all question a dermal structure, the enamel-organ an epithelial or epidermic structure. As I believe it can be shown that the enamel is formed by an actual conversion of the cells of the enamel-organ, this makes the dentine a dermal and the enamel an epidermic structure.

"6. In teleosts the new enamel-germs are formed directly from the oral epithelium. They are new formations, and arise quite independently of any portion of the germs of the teeth which preceded them. In mammals and reptiles, and in some of the batrachia, new tooth-germs are developed from portions of their predecessors.

"7. In all animals examined the phenomena are very uniform. A process dips in from the oral epithelium, often to a great depth, its end becoming transformed into an enamel-organ coincidentally with the formation of a dentine-papilla beneath it. The differences lie rather in such minor details as the extent to which a capsule is developed, and therefore no such generalization as that the teeth of fish in their development represent only an earlier stage of the development of the teeth of mammalia can be drawn."

Monsieur A. Chauveau's theory of the development of tooth-germs is as follows ("Comparative Anatomy of the Domesticated Animals," p. 921):

"The teeth are developed in the interior of a cavity, named the *dental follicle* or *sac*, by means of the elements of three germs, one belonging to the dentine, another to the enamel, and a third to the cement. The dental follicle is an oval cavity, with walls composed of two layers. The external is fibrous and complete; the internal, soft and gelatinous, is allied at the bottom to the dentine-germ. The latter is a prominence, which is detached from the bottom of the follicle, and has the exact shape of the tooth. Its structure comprises, in the center, delicate connective tissue, provided with vessels and nerves, and on the surface a layer of elongated cells. At the summit of the follicle, facing the dentine-germ, is the enamel-germ. It is exactly applied to the dentinal-pulp, which it invests like a cap, and is composed of a small mass of mucous connective tissue, covered by a layer of cylindrical cells, and joined to the buccal epithelium by the *gubernaculum dentis*.* According to Monsieur Magitot, the cement-organ manifestly exists in the foal. The base of the dentine-germ has been found, but it disappears rapidly after having performed its function.

"*Development of the Dental Follicle.*—On the free borders of the maxillæ, the epithelium of the buccal mucous membrane forms an elongated eminence—the *dental ridge*. Below this ridge the epithelium constitutes a bud, which develops in size, and is sunk in the mucous membrane. This is the enamel-germ. It has a layer of cylindrical cells on its deep surface, and in its center are round cells. After a certain time it is only joined to the epithelium, as already said, by a very thin line of cells, the *gubernaculum dentis*. While this enamel-germ grows downward, it covers, by its base, a connective bud which rises from the mucous derma. The two buds are reciprocally adapted to each other,

---

* Concerning the gubernaculum dentis Prof. C. S. Tomes says ("Dental Anatomy," p. 135): "Another structure, once thought to be important, but now known to be a mere bundle of dense fibrous tissue, is the 'gubernaculum.' The permanent tooth sacs, during their growth, have become invested by a bony shell, which is complete, save at a point near their apices, where there is a fora'men. Through this foramen passes a thin fibrous cord, very conspicuous when the surrounding bone is broken away, which is called the gubernaculum, from the notion entertained by the older anatomists that it was concerned in directing or effecting the eruption of the tooth. The gubernacula of the front permanent tooth sacs perforate the alveolus and blend with the gum behind the necks of the corresponding milk teeth, those of the bicuspids uniting with the periosteum of the alveoli of their deciduous predecessors."

and around them the connective tissue condenses and gives rise to the walls of the follicle. It will therefore be seen that the enamel-organ is a dependency of the epithelium, and the dentine-organ a production of the mucous derma.

"*Formation of the Dentine, Enamel, and Cement.*— As before said, the germ of the dentine has exactly the form of the future tooth; consequently the dentine which arises from its periphery presents the shape of a tooth also. The dentine and enamel are developed by the modification of the elements situated at the surface of their germs. The dentine is constituted of the cells of the germ, which send out ramifying and communicating prolongations—the *dentinal fibers*— and by an intercellular substance, which is impregnated with calcareous matter, and which, being molded around the fibers, forms canaliculi. The enamel is derived from the deep cells of its germ, which are elongated and prism-shaped, and are calcified in becoming applied to the surface of the dentine. The cement is developed at the expense of the walls of the follicle, according to the mode of ossification of the connective tissue.

"*Eruption.*—As the dentine is formed, the tooth increases in length and presses the enamel-germ upward. The latter, constantly compressed, becomes atrophied, and finally disappears when the tooth has reached the summit of the follicle. In the same way the young organ pierces the dental follicle and gum and makes its eruption externally.

"Such is the mode of the development of the temporary teeth, and the permanent ones are formed in the same manner. During the development of the germ of the temporary tooth, a bud is seen detaching itself from this germ and passing backward, to serve, at a later period, in forming the permanent tooth."

In another part of his work Prof. Chauveau says:

"The follicle in which the incisor teeth are developed shows only two papillæ. One, for the secretion of the dentine, is lodged in the internal cavity of the tooth, and is hollowed into a cup-shape at its free extremity; the other is contained in the external cul-de-sac."

In describing the simplicity of the structure of the horse's canine teeth (tushes), Prof. Lecoq says:

"The disposition of the developing follicle is in harmony with the simplicity of their structure. At the bottom there is a simple and conical papilla for the internal cavity; on the inner wall, a double longitudinal ridge, on which are molded the ridge and grooves on the inner face of the tooth."

Prof. William Youatt's theory of the development of horses' teeth is unique. He is probably correct about the bones or processes being separate, and his claim that they are solidified by the cement is certainly philosophical; but he differs from all other authorities about the enamel completing the formation of the tooth, for it is a well-known fact that a virgin tooth is enveloped by cement (its protecting varnish), which wears off as soon as the tooth is brought into use. He says ("The Horse," p. 223):

"A delicate membranous bag, containing a jelly-like substance, is found in a little cell within the jawbone of the unborn animal. It assumes by degrees the shape of the tooth, and then the jelly begins to change to bony matter. A hard and beautiful crystallization is formed on the membrane without, and so we have the cutting tooth covered by its enamel.

"In the formation of the grinders there are originally five membranous bags in the upper jaw and four in the lower. The jelly in them gives place to bony matter, which is supplied by little vessels, and which is represented by the darker portions of the cut with central black spots. The crystallization of enamel 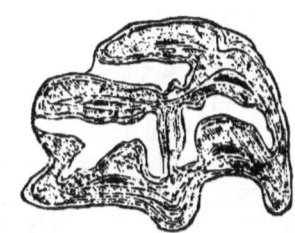 may be traced around each of the bags, and there would be five distinct bones or teeth but for the fact that a third substance is now secreted. (It is represented by the white spaces). It is a powerful cement, and through its agency the bones are united into one body, thus making one tooth of the five. This being done, another coat of enamel spreads over the sides, but not the top, and the tooth is completed."

Dr. Robley Dunglison's theory of the development of the human teeth is in principle the same as Prof. Youatt's theory regarding those of the horse. In his "Medical Dictionary," article "teeth," he says:

"The incisor and canine teeth are developed by a single point of ossification, the lesser molars by two, and the larger by four or five."

Surgeons M. H. Bouley and P. B. Ferguson believe that the teeth are the combined product of the secretion of the pulp and of the membrane which lines the alveolar cavities. They say that the question as to whether the sensibility of the teeth is inherent in the dental substance itself, or resides exclusively in the pulp, is a physiological point of which a satisfactory solution remains to be given.*

* Of the development of teeth in the human fetus Monsieur E. Magitot says ("Comtes Rendus," 1874): "*Seventh Week*— The epithelial eminence and epithelial inflection of Kölliker only may be seen at the edge of the jaw. The superior maxillary and intermaxillary bones are not united, and the inferior maxillary arch contains Meckel's cartilage only, without any trace of bone. The epithelial bands (enamel-organs) are successively formed in the order of their designation. *Ninth*—The dentine bulb appears in juxtaposition with the downward extremity of the enamel-organ. This stage occurs nearly simultaneously for the whole series of temporary follicles. *Tenth*— The wall of the follicle detaches itself from the base of the bulb and rises up its sides. *Fifteenth*—The epithelial band begins its transformation into an enamel-organ. The enamel-germ of the first *permanent* molar may now be seen springing from the epithelial inflection. *Sixteenth*—The wall of the follicle is closed. The epithelial band is broken, and the follicle thenceforward has no connection with the surface epithelium. The epithelial bands of the permanent teeth, which are derived from the necks of the enamel-organ of the corresponding deciduous teeth, appear. *Seventeenth*—Appearance of the cap of dentine of the central and lateral incisors; also the bulb of the first permanent molar. *Eighteenth*—Appearance of the dentine caps of the first and second molars; also the wall of the follicle of the permanent molar. *Twentieth*—Hight of the dentine caps of the central incisor, lateral incisor, and canine, .059; first and second molars, .039. Appearance of dentine organ of permanent teeth, and inclosure of wall and rupture of band of first molar. *Twenty-fifth*—Dentine caps, .07, .054. The permanent follicle walls, which appeared after the twenty-first week, have acquired a certain distinctness. *Twenty-eighth*—Dentine caps, .093, .078. The epithelial germs of the permanent follicles begin their transformation into enamel-organs: dentine cap first molar, .003 to .007. *Thirty-second*—Dentine caps, .113, .093. The first permanent molar cusps, which form upon the several apices of the dentine organ, have coalesced. *Thirty-sixth*—Dentine caps, .118, .109; permanent molar, .004 to .039. *Thirty-ninth*—Dentine caps, .136, .118; permanent molar, .039 to .073. The permanent follicle walls close. The dentine caps appear one month after birth."

# CHAPTER II.

### THE TEMPORARY DENTITION.

Twelve Incisors and Twelve Molars.—Why the Incisors are called "Nippers."—The Treatment of Foals Affects Teething.—Roots of Milk Teeth Absorbed by the Permanent.—The Tushes.

THE foal's temporary teeth (known also as milk or deciduous teeth) are adapted in size and number to the capacity of the jaws and the amount and nature of the mastication required for its sustenance. There are only twenty-four temporary teeth functionally developed. They consist of twelve incisors or nippers* and twelve molars or grinders, six above and six below of each kind. The dental formula is expressed thus:

$$\text{Incisors, } \tfrac{3}{3}-\tfrac{3}{3}; \text{ molars, } \tfrac{3}{3}-\tfrac{3}{3}=24.$$

According to Veterinary Dentist C. D. House, who says the care and treatment of foals will affect the growth of their teeth as much as they will their gen-

---

* Horsemen call the incisor teeth "Nippers." The word expresses the office they perform, to wit, nipping grass, as well as the word "grinder" does in the case of the molars—grinding corn. They call the first pair of incisors "central nippers," or "centrals," one being on either side of the median line; the second pair are the "dividers," for they stand between the first and third pairs; the third pair are called the "corners," from their forming the points of the crescent-like figure.

eral development, the foal has no teeth at birth, Nature providing a membrane-like cover for the incisors as well as the hoofs. In two or three days, however, the molars are all cut. The incisors are cut in pairs, two above and two below. The first pair protrude in from three to eight days, and attain their growth in about two months. The second pair are cut when the foal is five or six weeks old. They also attain their growth in about two months. The time of cutting the third pair varies. In some foals they appear as early as the sixth month; in others as late as the ninth. They attain their growth in about three months.*

The milk teeth are smaller and whiter and have more distinct necks than the permanent. Their shining, milky-white color, M. Chauveau says, is due to the thinness or absence of the cement, their crowns being finely striated (not cannular) on the anterior face, and their growth, unlike the permanent teeth, ceasing when they begin to be used.†

---

* M. Rousseau assigns from the seventh to the tenth month as the period of the completion of the first or colt's mouth dentition. The deciduous incisors have thinner and more trenchant crowns than the permanent.—*Owen.*

† The absorption of the roots of the milk teeth by the permanent would tend to prevent the continuous growth of the former; but the real cause appears to be that continuous growth is contrary to their nature. As the roots are composed of cement (except the dentine lining the pulp cavity), and as they are absorbed, it naturally follows that much of the cement surrounding the crowns of the permanent teeth is derived from them (cement from cement), thus lessening the drain on the permanent tooth pulps, which are all the better able to supply cement for the roots of the permanent teeth. The scarcity of cement on the crowns of the milk teeth is probably owing to the fact that they had no cement to absorb. The evil of extracting healthy milk teeth is obvious.

The incisors, which stand in an almost upright position, are smooth and rounded on the outer surface, but grooved on the inner. Their average length, including the root, is about an inch, their width about half an inch. The molars are about an inch and a quarter in length, and nearly an inch in long (antero-posterior) diameter. The short (transverse) diameter of the upper molars, which is about three-fourths of an inch, exceeds that of the lower nearly a half. Surgeon John Hughes says that in proportion to their length the breadth* of the temporary teeth is greater than the permanent. When first cut the incisor teeth are very sharp; the outer edges are higher than the inner, the slant resembling that of a chisel. A little wear, however, dulls the teeth, and brings the edges to a common level. The contrast between the edges of the corner incisors, however, is distinct for some time, the outer edge wearing off slowly.

There is a marked contrast in the appearance of the incisors at the age of one year and about the close of the second. At the former period they look new and fresh, standing close together, while at the latter they not only look old and worn, but the development of the jaws has caused them to stand apart. Their narrow necks are also conspicuous at two years of age.

The incisors are shed in the order in which they are cut. Nature provides them as they are needed, and takes them away so as to cause the least inconvenience to the foal. During the shedding of the central incisors foals have the use of the dividers and corners. The permanent centrals are ready for use before the dividers are shed, and the permanent dividers are

* "Breadth is antero-posterior diameter; thickness is transverse diameter."—*R. Owen*

ready before the corners are shed. However, during the shedding periods, particularly that of the central teeth, foals experience more or less difficulty in grazing; but if they are given a moderate quantity of soft, green food, their health will not be impaired, nor will they lose much flesh.

The central incisors are shed when the foal is about two years and a half old, the dividers at three and a half or four, and the corners at four and a half or five.

The molars, which Prof. Richard Owen says sooner begin to develop roots than the permanent, are shed with even less inconvenience to the foal than the incisors. The fourth grinder, the first permanent tooth cut, is ready for use before the first temporary molar is shed, and the fifth and sixth are ready before the second and third are shed. The time of shedding the twelve teeth varies somewhat, and the falling off of the "caps" of the uppers will precede those of the lower teeth several weeks. The caps are all that is left of the temporary molars, their roots and perhaps a small part of their bodies having been absorbed by the permanent. In most cases fully four-fifths of the crowns are worn off by attrition. Thus, when Nature is let alone, the temporary teeth are absorbed rather than shed; but when a shell is loose and in the way, it does no harm to remove it. The first molar is shed about the end of the second year, the second about the end of the third, and the third about the end of the fourth.

Surgeon W. A. Cherry says that the shedding of the teeth usually occurs in the Spring. There is, he says, a sufficient interval of time between the shedding of the upper and lower molars for the new teeth in the upper jaw to meet the old ones in the lower; sometimes the respective teeth, when the caps fall off, are not more than the sixteenth of an inch apart. He also says that as the temporary teeth wear down they become less and less dense.

While, as before said, it does no harm to remove loose shells, the punching out of a pair of incisors, which is sometimes done for the purpose of deception, frequently causes serious injury to the permanent pair (which should absorb the temporary, and fill the space that has become too large for it), not to mention the interference with grazing. The temporary teeth are often broken off at the neck and the sockets injured; this sometimes causes the permanent to grow irregularly, which in the case of the horse is a very serious matter, for if the permanent teeth do not meet, and are consequently not worn off by attrition, their growth, which continues throughout life, will cause trouble. There are cases, however, such as abnormal growths, accidents, &c., in which it is necessary to remove the temporary tooth, but the forceps only should be used. When the teeth have been removed for the purpose of deception, the object is to make it appear that they have been shed, and that the animal is older than it really is.

Veterinary authors, as a rule, do not mention the temporary tushes. A few odontologists, however, have described them. Prof. Owen ("Odontography," vol. i, p. 580) says "the small deciduous canine" is cut about the sixth month, at the time the third or corner incisors are cut. The lower tush, owing to its diminutive size, and its being so close to the incisor, "is shed almost as soon as the crown of the contiguous incisor is in full place, being carried out by the same movement." Bojanus,* Prof. Owen says, first "drew the attention of veterinary authors to it by his memoir 'De Dentibus Caninis Caducis,' &c. Bojanus never found the lower deciduous canine retained beyond the first year. The deciduous canine of the upper jaw, being developed at a short distance behind the incisors, is less disturbed by the eruption of the outer incisor, but is nevertheless shed in the course of the second year. The deciduous canines appear from Camper's † observations to retain their place longer in the zebra than in the horse."

Monsieur Lecoq says:

"The canine teeth are not shed, and grow but once. Some veterinarians, and among them Forthomme and Rigot, witnessed instances in which they were replaced; but the very rare exceptions cannot make us look upon these teeth as liable to be renewed. We must not, however, confound with these exceptionable cases the shedding of a small spicula or point, which, in the majority of horses, precedes the eruption of the real tusks."

Prof. C. S. Tomes says:

"The milk teeth of all the ungulata are very complete, and are retained late. They resemble the permanent teeth in general character, but the canines of the horse, as might have been expected—their greater development in the male being a sexual character—are rudimentary in the milk dentition."

* "Nova Acta Nat. Curios., tom. xii, part ii, p. 697. 1825."
† "Œuvres de Pierre Camper. Paris, 1805."

# CHAPTER III.

## THE PERMANENT DENTITION.

Distinction between Premolars and Molars.—The Bow-like Incisors.—Contrasts between the Upper and Lower Grinders, and the Rows formed by them.—The Incisors saved from Friction.—Horses' Teeth compared with those of other Animals.—Measurements.—Time's Changes.—Growth during Life.

THE Permanent Teeth, owing to their increased size and number, are as well adapted to the needs of the horse as the temporary are to the foal. In the males forty teeth are functionally developed;* in the females thirty-six, the latter, as a rule, having no canine teeth. However, their rudiments exist in the jaws, and sometimes, especially in old age, protrude. Of the forty teeth in the male horse there are twelve incisors, four canines or tushes (also called cannon or bridle teeth), twelve premolars,† and twelve molars. The dental formula is expressed thus:

$$I., \tfrac{3}{3}-\tfrac{3}{3}; \ C., \tfrac{1}{1}-\tfrac{1}{1}; \ P.M., \tfrac{3}{3}-\tfrac{3}{3}; \ M., \tfrac{3}{3}-\tfrac{3}{3} = 40.$$

---

\* The teeth that are not functionally developed are treated of in the chapter entitled "Remnant Teeth."

† "Premolars are teeth in front of the molars; they usually differ from them by being smaller and more simple in form, and in most animals have displaced deciduous predecessors. But they are not always smaller nor simpler in form (*e. g.,* the

The incisors and premolars absorb and replace the entire temporary dentition, except the shells or caps described in the preceding chapter, but the canines and molars are cut through the gums.

In veterinary works, as a rule, no distinction is made between a premolar and a molar, the twenty-four back teeth being called either molars or grinders. Prof. C. S. Tomes says the premolars and molars "are very similar to one another in shape, size, and in the pattern of their grinding surface." There is a difference, however, between the respective teeth, and naturalists make a distinction. The premolars (the three first back teeth), which replace the temporary molars, are slightly larger than the molars (the three last back teeth). They have besides a backward inclination, while the molars incline forward; the respective teeth are thus set *toward* one another. Both kinds are properly called grinders.

The permanent teeth are cut in pairs, two in either jaw, the upper teeth preceding the lower from one to two weeks. In the cutting of the canines, however, the reverse is the rule, for the lower teeth precede the upper. About a year's time elapses between the cutting of the respective pairs of teeth; that is, when the central incisors are cut, it will be about a year before the dividers will emerge. The rule is applicable to the premolars and molars also, but the case is different, for twenty-four of these teeth have to be cut during

horse); nor do they always displace deciduous predecessors (*e. g.*, they do not all do so in the marsupials); so that this definition is not absolutely precise. Still, as a matter of practice, it is usually easy to distinguish the premolars, and the division into premolars and molars is useful."—*C. S. Tomes,* "*Dental Anatomy,*" *&c., p. 258.*

the same period of time that the twelve incisors are cut. A permanent tooth attains its growth in about a year.

According to the best authorities, the molar and canine teeth are cut at the following periods: The first molars (in veterinary works they are called the *fourth*, because the three premolars come in front of them) are the first permanent teeth cut. The time of their cutting varies, for the foal's jaws must be sufficiently developed to afford them room, notwithstanding they are usually the smallest of the six back teeth. They are cut about the beginning of the second year, and are generally ready for use by the time the foal is two years old. The second molars are cut at about the age of two years, and are therefore fully developed by the end of the third year. The third pairs, the last of the molars, and consequently the most posterior of all the teeth, are sometimes cut as early as the third year, in which case they would be developed by the end of the third or the beginning of the fourth year. The time, however, may be prolonged six months or more. The canine teeth (tushes) emerge at or near the beginning of the fourth year.*

The time of the appearance of the incisors and premolars has already been indicated in the preceding chapter. However, the following extract from Prof. Owen's "Odontography" is appropriate in this place, as it throws further light on the subject, and to some extent agrees with the dates already given:

"The first true permanent molar appears between the eleventh and thirteenth months. The second fol-

---

* For further particulars concerning the tushes the reader is referred to the succeeding chapter.

lows between the fourteenth and twentieth months. The crowns of the premolars and the last true molar are now advancing in the closed sockets of reserve. The first premolar displaces the second,* and usually at the same time the very small deciduous molar, at from two years to two years and a half old. The first permanent incisor rises above the gum between two years and a half and three years. At the same period the second premolar pushes out the third deciduous molar. The last premolar displaces the last deciduous molar about the completion of the fourth year, and the appearance above the gum of the last true molar is usually anterior to this. The second incisor pushes out its predecessor between three and a half and four years. The small persistent canine or tusk, contrary to the usual rule, next follows, its development having received no check by the retention of its rudimental predecessor. Its appearance indicates the age of four years; but it sometimes appears earlier, rarely later. The third incisor pushes out the deciduous one about the fifth year, but is seldom completely in place before the horse is five years and a half old. The third premolars are then usually on a level with the other grinders."

On the completion of the fifth year a male foal is called a horse, a female or filly foal a mare. The teeth, however, are not all fully developed before the sixth year, and the roots of the grinders do not begin to

---

* To prevent confusion, it should be understood that Prof. Owen calls the "very small deciduous molar" here referred to the *first* deciduous molar, notwithstanding it is not functionally developed. Hence, as it has no successor, the *first* premolar displaces the *second deciduous* molar, the second premolar the third deciduous molar, and the third the fourth.

grow till about the seventh year, being, to use Prof. Owen's words, "implanted in the socket by an undivided base."

The incisor teeth, which will average about two inches and a quarter in length, are characterized by distinct curvatures, the outer surface, according to Surgeon John Hughes, forming a third of a circle, the inner a fifth. Were a string drawn from the crown of one of these teeth to the apex of the root, the figure would resemble a bow. The upper teeth are larger than the lower, and there is a difference in size of the respective teeth in both jaws, the centrals being larger than the dividers, and the dividers larger than the corners.

The incisors meet edge to edge, being thus admirably adapted for the purposes of grazing, and at the age of six years the bodies are nearly perpendicular one to the other. They form nearly semicircular figures, and, when the mouth is closed, present a rounded outer surface.

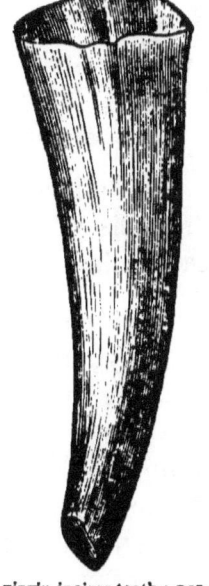

A virgin incisor tooth; posterior face.—*Chauveau.*

"The incisors," says Prof. Owen, "if found detached, recent or fossil, are distinguishable from those of the ruminants by their greater curvature, and from those of all other animals by the fold of enamel which penetrates the body of the crown, from its broad, flat summit, like the inverted finger of a glove."

The fold of enamel, which is commonly called the "mark," but which is also known as the infundibulum,

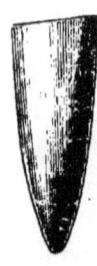

central enamel, &c., according to Surgeon J. Hughes's measurements, penetrates the lower centrals to the depth of from $\frac{3}{8}$ to $\frac{7}{10}$ of an inch; the dividers from $\frac{7}{10}$ to $\frac{4}{5}$, and the corners from $\frac{1}{4}$ to $\frac{3}{8}$. It penetrates the upper centrals from 1 inch and $\frac{1}{10}$ to 1 and $\frac{1}{2}$; the dividers from 1 and $\frac{1}{8}$ to 1 and $\frac{1}{4}$, and the corners from $\frac{4}{5}$ to nearly 1 inch. Prof. Youatt says the grinders have each two infundibula, which penetrate to their roots.

The following is Prof. A. Chauveau's description of the incisor teeth ("The Comparative Anatomy of the Domesticated Animals," Fleming's trans., p. 349):

"The general form of the incisors is that of a tri-faced pyramid, presenting an incurvation whose concavity is toward the mouth. The base of this pyramid, the crown of the tooth, is flattened before and behind. The summit or extremity of the fang, is, on the contrary, depressed on both sides. The shaft of the pyramid presents at different points of its hight, a series of intermediate conformations, which are utilized as indications of age, the continual growth of the teeth bringing each of them in succession to the frictional surface of the crown.

"Examined in a young tooth, but one that has completed its evolution, the free portion presents the following characteristics: An anterior face, indented by a slight longitudinal groove, which is prolonged to the root; a posterior face, rounded from side to side; two borders, of which the internal is always thicker than the external; and, lastly, the surface of friction. The latter does not exist in a tooth that has not been used, but in its stead are two sharp margins, circumscribing a cavity named the *external dental* cavity, or, better, *infundibulum*. This cavity terminates by a conical *cul-de-sac*, which descends more or less deeply into the substance of the tooth. The margins are designated the anterior and posterior. The latter, less elevated than the former, is cut by one or more notches, which are always deepest in the corner teeth. It is by the wear of these margins that the surface of friction is formed, and in the center of which the infundibulum persists during a certain period of time.

"The *root* is perforated by a single aperture, through which the pulp of the tooth penetrates into the internal cavity.

"In the composition of the incisor teeth are found the three fundamental substances of the dental organ. The *dentine* envelops the pulp cavity. Dentine is deposited in this cavity after the complete evolution of the tooth to replace the atrophied pulp, the yellow tint of which distinguishes it from the dentine of the first formation. It forms on the table of the tooth the mark designated by Girard the *dentinal star*.

"The *enamel* covers the dentine, not only on its free portion, but also on the roots; it does not extend, however, to their extremities. It is doubled into the external dental cavity, lining it throughout; and when the surface of friction is established, a ring of enamel may be seen surrounding it, and an internal ring circumscribing the infundibulum. The first circle is called the *encircling enamel*, the second the *central enamel*. In the virgin tooth the central enamel is continuous with the external enamel, and passes over the border which circumscribes the entrance to the infundibulum.

"The *cement* is applied over the enamel like a protecting varnish, but is not everywhere of the same thickness. On the salient portions it is extremely thin, and the friction caused by the food, the lips, and the tongue soon wears it away altogether. It is more abundant in depressed situations, as in the longitudinal groove on the anterior face of the tooth, and particularly at the bottom of the infundibulum. The quantity accumulated in this cul-de-sac is not, however, always the same. We have seen it almost null, and on the other hand, we possess an incisor unworn, or nearly so, in which the cavity is almost entirely obstructed by it. We are not aware that, up to the present time, any account has been taken of these differences in calculating the progress of wear; but it is manifest that they shorten or prolong the time required for the effacement of the infundibulum."

The grinder teeth, the horse's millstones, present various and interesting contrasts. They are separated from the incisors by a space that will average about four inches in extent, the sharp-pointed tushes (in males) only intervening. The space between the grinders and tushes is called the diastema (place for the bit). The upper grinders, except the first and last, are nearly quadrangular in form. The first and last, which exceed the others about a third of an inch in antero-posterior (front to rear) diameter, terminate in obtuse angles, which are far more pronounced on the inner than on the outer surface, thus affording the tongue fuller and freer play, without the danger of its being lacerated, as would be the case were the angles sharp. The form of the lower grinders, with the same exceptions in the case of the first and last, is nearly rectangular; their antero-posterior diameter is the same as that of the upper teeth, but their transverse diameter is nearly a half less.

The broad crowns of the upper teeth form what are called by veterinarians "tables," whereon the food is ground or kneaded by the narrow-crowned opposite grinders, the lateral movement of the lower jaw enabling the latter teeth to pass over the entire extent of the former.

The crown surfaces of the upper and lower rows are slanting instead of level, the former slanting inward, the latter outward. The inclined-planes are thus in perfect opposition, and yet in perfect harmony, for they facilitate the lateral and semicircular movement of the lower jaw during mastication.

The figures formed by the upper and lower rows of grinders, aside from the difference in their thickness, are very dissimilar. The upper rows are slightly concave, and converge in conformity to the narrowing of the jaws; the space between the sixth grinders averages about two inches and four-fifths, while that between the first is about two inches. The lower rows form regular but oblique lines, which also converge, like the sides of a hopper, in conformity to the narrowing of the jaws, the space between the two sixth grinders and the two first averaging respectively two inches and a half and one inch and a half. Thus, when the mouth is closed, the lower teeth in the region of the sixth grinders scarcely cover a third of the crown surface of the upper teeth, while those in the region of the first barely lap their inner edges. This apparent structural defect is overcome by the lateral movement of the lower jaw, which, owing to the fact that it increases in proportion to the distance from its hinge-like joint in the region of the temporal bone and zygomatic arch,* is greater in the region of the first grinders than in that of the sixth. Therefore it will be perceived that it is only alternately that the rows are used in the performance of the masticatory function, and that were the grinders in exact apposition (edge to edge), the lateral and semicircular movement of the lower jaw would be as awkward and unnatural in the case of the horse as the same movement would be in a human being.

There are still other contrasts between the grinders. According to Surgeons M. H. Bouley and P. B. Ferguson, the upper teeth are slightly convex, the lower slightly concave. Again, according to Charles D. House, the outer surface of the upper grinders is provided with a coat of enamel twice as thick as that of the inner, while the reverse is the case with the lower teeth. There is design in this provision of Nature (notwithstanding Mr. House says it is inexplicable), for the projecting edges receive that which they require, to wit, strength in proportion to their hight; otherwise they would be easily broken off. As the

---

* Prof. Youatt says: "The branches of the lower jaw terminate in two processes, the coracoid (beak-like), and the condyloid (rounded). The coracoid passes under the zygomatic arch, the temporal muscle being inserted into it and wrapped round it. The condyloid is received into the glenoid (shallow) cavity of the temporal bone, at the base of the zygomatic arch, and forms the joint on which the lower jaw moves. The joint admits of a hinge-like motion, which is the action of the jaw in nipping the herbage and seizing the corn. The corn, however, must be ground; bruising and champing it are not sufficient for the purposes of digestion. It must be put into a mill. It *is* put into a mill, and as perfect a one as imagination can conceive. The construction of the glenoid cavity gives the required lateral or grinding motion."

lower edges have only about half the hight of the upper, they do not require more than half the quantity of enamel to strengthen them. Another use of this unequal disposition of enamel is its tendency, by its wear, to preserve the slant of the respective crown surfaces. Further, the dentine, which fills the interspaces between the folds or ridges of enamel, being softer than the enamel, wears out faster, thus keeping the ridges sharp.* The grinders are therefore, owing to this "interblending of the dental tissues," their own whetstones as well as the horse's millstones.

Some writers, even of the present day, deny that the enamel penetrates to the interior of the grinders; but the fact that it does was established by John Hunter over a century ago, and a cut of a section of a horse's grinder (slightly magnified) showing the enamel folds,

---

* Prof. R. Owen illustrates the above principle in the Introduction to his "Odontography," page 26. He says: "It (the enamel) sometimes forms only a partial investment of the crown, as in the molar teeth of the iguanodon, the canine teeth of the hog and hippopotamus, and the incisors of the Rodentia. In these the enamel is placed only on the front of the tooth, but is continued along a great part of the invested base, which is never contracted into one or divided into more roots, so that the character of the crown of the tooth is maintained throughout its extent as regards both its shape and structure. The partial application of the enamel operates in maintaining a sharp edge upon the exposed and worn end of the tooth precisely as the hard steel keeps up the outer cutting edge of the chisel by being welded against an inner plate of softer iron."

Prof. C. S. Tomes, speaking of the grinder teeth of the horse, says: "As each ridge and pillar of the tooth consists of dentine bordered by enamel, and the arrangement of the ridges and pillars is complex, and as, moreover, cementum fills up the interspaces, it is obvious that an efficient rough grinding surface will be preserved by the unequal wear of the several tissues."

may be found in his "Natural History of the Human Teeth."

The formation of the enamel is thus described by Prof. Bouley and Surgeon Ferguson ("Veterinarian," 1844):

"In the grinder teeth the enamel may be said to resemble a little ribbon, which forms, in refolding many times upon itself in the interior of the tooth, a succession of undulating planes, and constitutes the hard external envelop of the cubic mass of the organ. An idea of this disposition may be formed on examining a tooth which is not yet cut, but which is ready to be cut. Those that have been worn, present on their crowns, besides the undulating lines of the enamel envelop, a succession of reliefs, salient and sinuous, of the substance of the enamel, which are nothing else than the free borders of this folded ribbon. It is in the intervals of the folds of enamel that is deposited the ivory-colored substance (dentine), which renders the tooth a solid mass when it has attained its full growth."

Prof. Richard Owen, one of the first odontologists of the age, in whose numerous works descriptions of many kinds of teeth may be found, has paid a fair share of attention to the study of horses' teeth, both recent and fossil. His description of the grinders and comparisons with the teeth of other animals are too interesting to be omitted here, and render any apology for the few repetitions of facts already given unnecessary. He says ("Odontography," vol. i, p. 572):

"The horse will yield us the first example of the dentition of the hoofed quadrupeds with toes in uneven number, because it offers in this part of its organization some transitional features between the dental characters of the typical members of the isodactyle and of those of the anisodactyle ungulata.

"All the kinds of teeth are retained and in almost normal numbers in both jaws, with as little unequal or excessive development as in the anoplothere,* but the prolongation of the slender jaws carries the canines and incisors to some distance from the grinders, and creates a long diastema, as in the ruminants† and tapirs.‡

---

* "The anoplothere was one of the earliest forms of hoofed quadrupeds introduced upon the surface of this earth, and it is characterized by the most complete system of dentition. It not only possessed incisors and canines in both jaws, but they were so equally developed that they formed one unbroken series with the premolars and molars, which character is now found only in the *human species*. The dental formula is: I., 3—3, 3—3; C., 1—1, 1—1; P. M., 4—4, 4—4; M., 3—3, 3—3=44. The Anoplothere Commune was the size of an ass, and, with the other species of the extinct genus, had a cloven hoof, like the Ruminants, but the division extended through the metacarpus and metatarsus. The anoplothere was an animal of aquatic habits, and had a very long and strong tail, which Cuvier conjectures to have been used like that of the otter in swimming."—*Owen*.

† "The ordinary dental formula of the Ruminantia is: I. (upper jaw), 0—0, (lower jaw), 3—3; C., 0—0, 1—1; P. M., 3—3, 3—3; M., 3—3, 3—3=32. The antelopes, the sheep, and the ox, which are collectively designated the 'hollow-horned' ruminants, present this formula. It likewise characterizes many of the 'solid-horned' ruminants, or the deer tribe, the exceptions having canine teeth in the upper jaw in the male sex, and sometimes also in the female, though they are always smaller in the latter."—*Owen*.

‡ "The dental formula of the tapir is: I., 3—3, 3—3; C., 1—1, 1—1; P. M., 4—3, 4—3; M., 3—3, 3—3=42."—*Owen*.

It is noteworthy that the dentition of the tapir corresponds precisely in number with that of the horse, provided the latter's

"The upper grinder teeth present a modification of the complex structure intermediate between the anoplotherian and ruminant patterns. The crown is cubical, but is impressed on the outer surface by two wide and deep longitudinal channels. It is penetrated from within by a valley, which enters obliquely from behind forward. This is crossed by two crescentic valleys, which soon become insulated, as in the camel;* but a large internal lobe, at the end of the oblique valley, presents more of the anoplotherian proportions than is shown by any ruminant. It is at first distinct; but although it soon becomes confluent with the anterior lobe in the existing species of the horse, it continued distinct much longer, and with more of the conical or columnar form, in the primigenial horse of the miocene tertiary period.

"The grinder teeth of the horse, Cuvier† remarks,

---

Remnant teeth are counted; and, besides, the odd teeth in both animals appear in the *upper* jaw. Prof. T. H. Huxley says: "Deepen the valley, increase the curvature of the (outer) wall and lam'inæ (transverse ridges); give the latter a more directly backward slope; cause them to develop accessory ridges and pillars, and the upper molars of the tapir will pass through the structure of that of the rhinoceros to that of the horse."

* "The dental formula of the camel is: I., 1—3, 1—3; M., 6—6, 6—6=32. The anterior molars are conical. They are separated from the posterior molars, and are sometimes regarded as canines. The upper incisors are also conical, compressed, somewhat curved, resembling canines, and are used for tearing up the hard and strong plants of the desert, on which the animal usually feeds."—*American Cyclopedia*.

† A French naturalist. Died May 13, 1832. "He is regarded as the founder of the science of comparative anatomy, and his knowledge of the science was such that a bone or a small fragment of a fossil animal enabled him to determine the order, and

have a closer analogy with those of the rhinoceros\*
than might at first be supposed. The anterior crescentic enamel represents the termination of the principal or oblique valley, which is cut off by a bridge of dentine analogous to that in the leptorhine rhinoceros. The posterior crescentic island is a further development of the folds in the rhinoceros' molar, but is much earlier insulated in the horse.

"In the lower jaw the same analogies may be traced. The teeth, on the outer side, are divided into two convex lobes by a median longitudinal fissure; on the inner side they present three principal unequal convex ridges, and an anterior and posterior narrower ridge. The crown of the grinder is penetrated from the inner side by deeper and more complex folds than in the anoplothere, and still more so than in the rhinoceros

even genus, to which it belonged. The time of Cuvier marks the opening of a new epoch in comparative anatomy. He applied this science to natural history, physiology, and to the study of fossils The first edition of "Leçons d'Anatomie Comparée" appeared about the beginning of the present century, and the second was the last work upon which Cuvier labored. For more than thirty years he had collected an immense amount of facts and materials, which are partly embodied in this book. It is a monument of patient industry, a model in arrangement, and a mine of knowledge, of which all observers since have availed themselves."—*American Cyclopedia.*

\* "The essential characteristics of the dentition of the genus rhinoceros are to be found in the form and structure of the molar teeth. They differ essentially from those of the horse by being implanted by distinct roots. The normal dental formula of the molar series is: P. M., 4—4, 4—4; M., 3—3, 3—3=28. There are no canines. As to the incisors, the species vary, not only in regard to their form and proportions, but also their existence."—*Owen.*

and paleothere.* The anterior valley between the narrow ridge and the first principal internal column expands into a subcrescentic fold. The second is a short, simple fold, and terminates opposite that which penetrates the tooth from the outer side. The third inner fold expands in the posterior lobe of the tooth like the first, and two short folds partially detach a small accessory lobe at the posterior part of the crown. All the valleys, fissures, or folds, in both the upper and the lower grinders, are lined by enamel, which also coats the whole exterior surface of the crown.

"The character by which horses' grinders may best be distinguished from the teeth of other herbivora corresponding with them in size, is the great length of the tooth before it divides into roots. This division, indeed, does not begin to take place until much of the crown has been worn away. Thus, except in old horses, a considerable proportion of the whole of the tooth is implanted in the socket by an undivided base. This is slightly curved in the upper grinders.

"The deciduous molars have shorter bodies than the permanent, and sooner begin to develop roots. They may be distinguished from the rooted molar of a ruminant, as may also their permanent successors with roots, by their form and the pattern of their grinding surface. The latter may be a little changed by the partial obliteration of its enamel folds, but it generally retains enough of its character to show the distinction."

* "The species of paleotherium, which appear to have accompanied the anoplotheres in the first introduction of hoofed quadrupeds upon this planet, were characterized by the same complete dental formula, namely, forty-four functionally developed teeth."—*Owen.*

Monsieur Lecoq's description of the grinder teeth, like the one just quoted, is a contribution to dental science. The repetition of facts already given is offset by its additional facts, and its historical information is as interesting as are Prof. Owen's comparisons. It is as follows ("Traité de l'Exterieur du Cheval et des Principaux Animaux Domestiques") :

"It was believed for a long time that the grinders of Solipeds were all persistent teeth. This error, founded on the authority of Aristotle, was so deeply rooted that, although Ruini, toward the end of the Sixteenth century, had discovered the existence of two temporary molars, Bourgelat did not believe it when he founded the French veterinary schools, and was only convinced when Tenon proved by specimens, in 1770, that the first three are deciduous.

"Generally considered, the grinder arcades have not the same disposition in both jaws. Wider apart in the superior one, they form a slight curve, whose convexity is outward. In the inferior jaw, on the contrary, the two arcades separate in the form of a V toward the back of the mouth. Instead of coming in contact by level surfaces, the grinders meet by inclined-planes. In the lower jaw the internal border is higher than the external, while the reverse is the rule in the upper. This circumstance prevents the lateral movement of the lower jaw taking place without separation of the incisors, and thus saves them from friction.

"Like the incisors, each grinder presents for study a free and a fixed portion. The free portion (the body), nearly square in the upper grinders, broader than thick in the lower, shows at the external surface of the former two longitudinal grooves, the anterior of which is the deeper, both being continued on the incased portion. This is not the case with the lower grinders, which have but one narrow and frequently indistinct groove. The internal surface, in both jaws, presents only one groove, and that but little marked. It is placed backward in the upper teeth, and is most apparent toward the root. The anterior and posterior faces of the respective teeth, which are in contact with each other, are nearly level, but at the extremities of the arcades the isolated faces are converted into a narrow border.

"The grinders are separated from each other by their imbedded portion, particularly at the extremities of the arcades, an arrangement which strengthens them by throwing the strain put upon the terminal teeth toward the middle of the line. They exhibit a variety of roots. In the first and last, either above or below, there are three, while the intermediate teeth have four in the upper jaw, and only two in the lower. The root, if examined a short time after the eruption of the free portion, looks only like the shaft of the latter, without fangs,* but a wide internal cavity. The roots form when the teeth begin to be pushed from their sockets; they cease to grow as soon as their cavities are filled with new dentine, but the tooth, constantly growing, causes the walls inclosing it to contract; so that in extreme age the shaft, completely worn away, leaves several stumps formed by the roots.

"The replacement of the twelve molars is not at all like what happens with the incisors. They grow im-

---

* Fang for *root* is obsolete. Fang signifies *crown*—especially the pointed teeth of animals of prey and the poison-fang of serpents. Fang for both root and crown causes confusion.

mediately below the temporary teeth, and divide their two roots into four, the absorbing process continuing until the bodies are reduced to simple plates and fall off."

In measuring the teeth in a large-sized head the following facts and figures were elicited: Length of grinder rows, 7 inches. Space between the sixth grinders, upper rows, measuring from the inner surfaces, but not including the angles, 3 inches; center of rows, $2\frac{3}{16}$; first grinders, not including the space of the angles, $2\frac{1}{16}$. Lower rows: Between the sixth grinders, $2\frac{5}{8}$; center of rows, $1\frac{5}{16}$; first grinders, $1\frac{1}{2}$. Upper tush from first grinder, $2\frac{3}{8}$; from third incisor, $1\frac{1}{8}$. Lower tush from grinder, $3\frac{1}{2}$; from incisor, $\frac{5}{8}$. Space between the upper tushes, 2; between the lower, $1\frac{3}{4}$. Space between the upper corner incisors, measuring from center of teeth, 2; lower, $1\frac{5}{16}$; between the upper dividers, $1\frac{1}{2}$; lower, $1\frac{3}{8}$. Distance around semicircle of upper incisors, $4\frac{7}{16}$; around lower, $3\frac{11}{16}$.

As a supplement to the above, the following extract is made from "An Essay on the Teeth" by Surgeon John Hughes ("Veterinarian," 1841, "Proceedings Vet. Med. Ass.," p. 22):

"The upper and lower grinders will measure from $2\frac{1}{2}$ to 3 inches in length. In transverse diameter the former exceed the latter in the proportion of 7 to 4. The aggregate measurement of the sockets of the upper grinders is about 7 inches. The first tooth occupies one inch and a half of this space, the second $1\frac{1}{4}$, the third $1\frac{1}{8}$, the fourth 1, the fifth 1, and the sixth $1\frac{1}{4}$. The breadth of the corresponding lower teeth is about the same as that of the upper."

There is a difference in the structure of all the teeth, and an expert can tell to which socket each belongs. They fit their sockets accurately,* are braced all round by the jawbone processes, and receive besides support and protection from the gums, which adhere to them tenaciously and are almost as hard as cartilage. Use and time, however, work changes, the teeth all wearing down, the incisors in particular changing shape and projecting outward. At the age of twelve years the gums begin to slacken, causing the teeth to look longer. The change from the upright position of the incisors, and the increased space between them and the canines, is caused by the elongation of the jaws, which carries the incisors outward. The canines do not change their position, but they become mere stubs.

* "The manner of attachment of the human teeth is that termed 'gomphosis,' *i. e.*, an attachment comparable to the fitting of a peg into a hole. The bony sockets, however, allow of a considerable degree of motion, as may be seen by examining the teeth in a dried skull, the fitting being in the fresh state completed by the interposition of the dense periosteum of the socket. This latter, by its elasticity, allows of a small degree of motion in the tooth, and so doubtless diminishes the shock which would be occasioned by mastication were the teeth perfectly immovable and without a yielding lining within their sockets."—*C. S. Tomes, "Dental Anatomy," &c., p. 23.*

John Hunter says ("Human Teeth"): "The roots of the teeth are fixed in the gum and alveolar processes by that species of articulation called *gomphosis*, which in some measure resembles a nail driven into a piece of wood. They are not, however, firmly united with the processes, for every tooth has some degree of motion; and in heads which have been boiled or macerated in water, so as to destroy the periosteum and adhesion of the teeth, we find them so loosely connected with their sockets that the incisors are ready to drop out, the grinders remaining, as it were, hooked, from the number and shape of their roots."

Notwithstanding all these changes it is a rare thing to see a missing incisor or grinder. The canines, however, owing perhaps to their sharp points, not only wear out, but now and then, in extreme old age, fall out.

The permanent teeth agree with the temporary in but few respects, though the general appearance of the respective teeth is nearly the same. They differ in many respects. Their bodies are larger and denser, and their roots longer and stronger. The grooving of the incisors is the reverse; the outer surface is usually double grooved, the inner smooth, both being slightly rounded. They are less upright in position, and less sharp, but are more discolored, and the "marks" (infundibula) are wider and deeper and wear out more slowly. They attain their growth more slowly, and a healthy tooth continues to grow throughout life.

In proof of the last assertion many authorities could be cited, but those that follow must suffice. It is a wise provision of Nature, as but for it a horse's teeth, particularly the grinders, would be worn to stubs in two or three years after their development. Prof. M. H. Bouley and Surgeon P. B. Ferguson say ("Veterinarian," 1844):

"The growth throughout life is a compensation for the enormous wear of the teeth, the horse having to perform for himself that which the miller performs for man; and thus during a very long time the teeth preserve, if not their form, at least their length."

Prof. A. Chauveau, referring to the horse, says:

"The permanent teeth present in their development a common but very remarkable characteristic, rarely met with in other animals. They are thrust up from the alveoli during the entire life of the animal to replace the surface worn by friction."

The activity of the growth of the grinders is remarkable about the seventh year, for at this time their roots begin to develop; growth is thus going on at both ends at the same time. A third movement is now at least apparent, for the undivided base in the socket appears to be slowly pushed out, which may partly account for the shrinkage of the gums. The tenacity of the adhesion of the *periosteum* would not wholly prevent this movement, for it acts as a *cushion*, its elasticity preventing concussions. The undivided base resembles a post set in the ground, except that the implanted part is smaller than the crown.

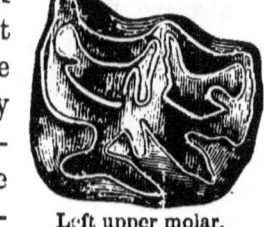

Left upper molar.

Up to about the sixteenth year, the growth of the teeth results chiefly from vitality transmitted through the medium of the pulp. After the pulp has become converted into dentine, however, the tooth " draws its nourishment from the blood-vessels of the socket." *

Surgeon Louis Brandt (" The Age of Horses," Indianola, Texas, 1860) says of the incisors :

"The length of the teeth is constantly decreasing, and often quite regularly, so that in extreme old age they will sometimes not exceed half an inch in length, while at their prime they were 2¼ to 3 inches long. Their breadth decreases nearly in proportion to the decrease in length."

\* See pages 169–70.

## CHAPTER IV.

### THE CANINE TEETH OR TUSHES.

**Practically Useless.**—Different in their Nature from the other Teeth.—Were they formerly Weapons of Offense and Defense?—Views of Messrs. Darwin, Hunter, Bell, Youatt, and Winter.—Their time of Cutting the most Critical Period of the Horse's Life.

THE Canine Teeth (*laniarii dentes*), comparatively speaking, are of little practical use; at least they are of little use to the modern horse. They have been much reduced in size during the evolution of the horse, and, if Mr. C. R. Darwin's theory is correct, are probably "in the course of ultimate extinction." They distinguish the sex, it is true, but their loss would not be felt on that account. The horse sometimes uses them in tearing bark from trees, for he is by instinct his own (botanical) doctor, and the bark is his medicine. The sharp points of the tushes penetrate the bark more readily than the incisors, and apparently the horse wishes to save his incisors, thus showing his horse-sense. Their nature is different from that of the other teeth, for the incisors and grinders grow till old age. This is not the case with the tushes, and, further, they are never in apposition (superposed), and consequently do not wear one another.

The lower tushes, as before said, are about three-fourths of an inch from the corner incisors, and about three inches and a half from the first grinders. The space between the upper tushes and the corner incisors is double that of the lower, and they are consequently three-fourths of an inch nearer the grinders. The distances may vary a half an inch or more. The space between the tushes and grinders is, as already said, called the diastema.

The average hight of the tushes when full grown is about three-fourths of an inch. They resemble triangles, having broad bases and sharp crowns, the latter being remarkable, says Prof. Owen, "for the folding in of the anterior and posterior margins of enamel, which here includes an extremely thin layer of dentine." They have a slight outward inclination, that of the lower teeth exceeding that of the upper. Their outer surface is oval, the inner (in the young horse) being deeply grooved. As age advances the inner surface becomes oval also, and the crowns more or less blunt. The root of a tush, which is longer than its body, has a distinct backward curvature, rendering the extraction of these teeth almost impossible. The tushes have no "marks" (infundibula), the nerve cavity extending through nearly the entire length of the tooth.

Monsieur Lecoq says:

"The free portion of the tusk, slightly curved and thrown outward, particularly in the lower jaw, presents two faces (internal and external), separated from one another by two sharp borders, which incline to the inner side, and meet in a point at the extremity of the tooth. The external face, slightly rounded, presents a series of fine striæ, longitudinal and parallel. The internal has a conical eminence in its middle, whose point is directed toward that of the tooth, and is separated from each border by a deep groove.

"The root of the tusk, more curved than the free portion, bears internally a cavity analogous to that of the root of the incisors, and, like it, diminishes in size and finally disappears as age advances; but it is always relatively larger, because of the absence of the infundibulum in the canine teeth.

"The structure of these teeth is much simpler than that of the incisors, consisting, as they do, of a central mass of dentine, hollowed by the pulp cavity, and covered by an external layer of enamel, on which is deposited a little cement."

As there is more or less mystery about the tushes, and as they are important factors in the consideration of the problem of the evolution of the horse as well as other animals, a few extracts from the works of well-known scientific men, giving their views on the subject, will prove interesting if not instructive.

Mr. Charles R. Darwin gives the following interesting account of tushes and their uses in certain animals, among them the horse ("Descent of Man," vol. ii, pp. 245-6-7):

" Male quadrupeds which are furnished with tusks use them in various ways, as in the case of horns. The boar strikes laterally and upward, the musk-deer with serious effect downward. The walrus, though having a short neck and unwieldy body, 'can strike upward, downward, or sideways with equal dexterity.' The Indian elephant fights, as I was informed by the late Dr. Falconer, in a different manner according to the position and curvature of his tusks. When they are directed forward and upward, he is able to fling a tiger to a great distance—it is said to even thirty feet;

when they are short and turned downward, he endeavors suddenly to pin the tiger to the ground, and in consequence is dangerous to the rider, who is liable to be dismounted.

"Very few male quadrupeds possess weapons of two distinct kinds specially adapted for fighting with rival males. The male muntjac-deer (*Cervulus*), however, offers an exception, as he is provided with horns and exserted canine teeth. But one form of weapon has often been replaced in the course of ages by another form, as we may infer from what follows. With ruminants the development of horns generally stands in an inverse relation with that of even moderately well-developed canine teeth. Thus camels, guanacoes, chevrotains, and musk-deer are hornless, and they have efficient canines, these teeth being 'always of smaller size in the females than in the males.' Male deer and antelopes, on the other hand, possess horns, and they rarely have canine teeth, and these when present are always of smaller size, so that it is doubtful whether they are of any service in their battles. With *Antelope montana* they exist only as rudiments in the young male, disappearing as he grows old. Stallions have small canine teeth, but they do not appear to be used in fighting, for stallions bite with their incisors, and do not open their mouths widely like camels and guanacoes. Whenever the adult male possesses canines now in an inefficient state, while the female has either none or mere rudiments, we may conclude that the early male progenitor of the species was provided with efficient canines, which had been partially transferred to the females. The reduction of these teeth in the males seems to have followed from some change in their manner of fighting, often caused (but not in the case of the horse) by the development of new weapons."

In the first volume of the "Descent of Man," page 139, Mr. Darwin attributes the reduction in size of the tushes in horses to their " habit of fighting with their incisor teeth and hoofs," and on page 231, of the second volume, he continues the discussion of canines in different animals as follows:

" In the male dugong the upper incisors form offensive weapons. In the male narwhal one of the upper teeth is developed into the well-known, spirally-twisted, so-called horn, which is sometimes from nine to ten feet long. It is believed that the males use these horns for fighting together, for 'an unbroken one can hardly be got, and occasionally one may be found with the point of another jammed into the broken place.' The tooth on the opposite side of the head in the male consists of a rudiment about ten inches in length, which is imbedded in the jaw. It is not, however, very uncommon to find double-horned male narwhals in which both teeth are well developed. In the females both teeth are rudimentary. The male cach'alot* has a

* "Sperm-whale or cachalot (*Physeter macrocephalus*). My friend Mr. Broderip possesses a tooth of a male Physeter, with the base open and uncontracted, which measures nine inches and a half in length, nine inches in circumference, and weighs three pounds. An ingenious whale-fisher has carved the chief incidents of his exciting and dangerous occupation on one side of this very fine tooth. The other side bears the following inscription: 'The tooth of a sperm-whale, that was caught by the ship Adam's crew, off Albemarle Point, and made 100 bbls. of oil, in the year 1817.' Below the inscription are two excellent figures of the cachalot, one spouting, the other dead and marked for flensing."—*Owen's "Odontography," Vol. I, pp 353-4.*

larger head than the female, and it no doubt aids these animals in their aquatic battles. Lastly, the adult male ornithorhyn'chus is provided with a remarkable apparatus, namely, a spur on the foreleg, closely resembling the poison fang of a venomous snake. Its use is not known, but we may suspect it serves as a weapon of offense. It is represented by a mere rudiment in the female."*

The foregoing extracts would not be complete without giving the views of this great disciple of evolution concerning the same teeth in man. He says ("Descent of Man," vol. i, p. 198):

"We have thus far endeavored rudely to trace the genealogy of the vertebrata by the aid of their mutual affinities. We will now look to man as he exists, and we shall, I think, be able partially to restore during successive periods, but not in due order of time, the structure of our early progenitors. This can be effected by means of the rudiments which man still retains, by the characters which occasionally make their appearance in him through reversion,† and by the aid of the principles of morphology and embryology.‡ The early

---

* For further information concerning this strange animal see the "Vocabulary."

† "The occasional appearance at the present day of canine teeth which project above the others, with traces of a diastema or open space for the reception of the opposite canines, is in all probability a case of reversion to a former state, when the progenitors of man were provided with these weapons."—"*Descent of Man,*" Vol. II, p. 309.

‡ "The human em'bryo resembles in various points of structure certain low forms when adult. For instance, the heart at first exists as a simple pulsating vessel; the excreta are voided through a cloacal passage, and the os coccyx projects like a true

progenitors of man were no doubt once covered with hair, both sexes having beards. Their ears were pointed and capable of movement, and their bodies were provided with a tail, having the proper muscles. Their limbs and bodies were also acted on by muscles which now only occasionally reappear, but are normally present in the quadrumana. The great artery and

tail, 'extending considerably beyond the rudimentary legs.' The great-toe, as Prof. Owen remarks, 'which forms the fulcrum when standing or walking, is perhaps the most characteristic peculiarity in the human structure;' but in an embryo about an inch in length, Prof. Wyman found that the great-toe was shorter than the others, and instead of being parallel to them, 'projected at an angle from the side of the foot, thus corresponding with the permanent condition of this part in the quadrumana.' * * * When the extremities are developed, 'the feet of lizards and mammals, the wings and feet of birds, no less than the hands and feet of man, all arise from the same fundamental form.' (Von Baer)."—"*Descent of Man,*" *Vol. I, pp. 14–16.*

"Each human individual is developed from an egg, and this egg is a simple cell, like that of any animal or plant. The embryo, in the early stages of development, is not at all different from those of other animals. At a certain period it has essentially the anatomical structure of a lancelet (the lowest vertebrate), later of a fish, and in subsequent stages those of amphibian and mammal forms. In the further evolution of these mammal forms, those first appear which stand lowest in the series, namely, forms allied to beaked animals (ornithorhynchus); then those allied to pouched animals (marsupials), which are followed by forms most resembling apes, till at last the peculiar human form is produced as the final result. Every one knows that the butterfly proceeds from a pupa, the pupa from a caterpillar, to which it bears no resemblance, and again the caterpillar from the egg of the butterfly. But few, except those of the medical profession, are aware that man, in the course of his individual evolution, passes through a series of transformations

nerve of the humerus ran through a supra-condyloid fora'men. At this or some earlier period the intestine gave forth a much larger diverticulum or cæcum than that now existing. The foot, judging from the condition of the great-toe in the fetus, was then prehensile, and our early progenitors were no doubt arboreal in their habits, frequenting some warm, forest-clad land. The males were provided with great canine teeth, which served them as formidable weapons."\*

no less astonishing and remarkable than the well known metamorphoses of the butterfly. \* \* \* An examination of the human embryo in the third or fourth week of its evolution shows it to be altogether different from the fully developed man, and that it exactly corresponds to the undeveloped embryo-form presented by the ape, the dog, the rabbit, the horse, and other mammals, at the same stage of their ontog'eny (germ history), which may be demonstrated by placing the respective embryos side by side. At this stage it is a bean-shaped body of very simple structure, with a tail behind, and two pairs of paddles, resembling the fins of fish, and totally dissimilar at the sides to the limbs of man and other mammals. Nearly the whole of the front half of the body consists of a shapeless head, without a face, on the sides of which are seen gill-fissures and gill-arches, as in fishes. \* \* \* The human embryo passes through a stage in which it possesses no head, no brain, no skull; in which the trunk is still entirely simple and undivided into head, neck, breast, and abdomen, and in which there is no trace of arms or legs."—*Ernst Heinrich Haeckel*, "*The Evolution of Man*," *Vol. I, pp. 3, 18, 253.*

\* Mr. Darwin continues: "At a much earlier time the uterus was double; the excreta were voided through a cloaca, and the eye was protected by a third eyelid or nictitating membrane. At a still earlier period the progenitors of man must have been aquatic in their habits, for morphology plainly tells us that our lungs consist of a modified swim-bladder, which once served as a float. The clefts on the neck in the embryo of man show where the branchiæ once existed," &c., &c.

Again, on page 138 of the same volume, Mr. Darwin says:

"The early progenitors of man were, as previously stated, probably furnished with great canine teeth; but as they gradually acquired the habit of using stones, clubs, or other weapons for fighting with their enemies, they would have used their jaws and teeth less and less. In this case the jaws and the teeth would have become reduced in size, as we may feel sure from numerous analogous cases."*

Dr. John Hunter, writing nearly one hundred years before Mr. Darwin's time, says ("The Human Teeth," p. 29):

"The use of the cuspidati would seem to be to lay hold of substances, perhaps even living animals. They are not formed for dividing, as the incisors are, nor are they fit for grinding. We may trace in these teeth a similarity in shape, situation, and use, from the most imperfectly carnivorous animal—which we believe to be the human species—to the most perfectly carnivorous, namely, the lion."

The editor of Dr. Hunter's work, Mr. Thomas Bell, F.R.S., comments as follows on the above extract:

"That our conclusions as to the functions of an organ as it exists in man, when drawn exclusively from analogous structures in the lower animals, will fre-

---

* "The jaws, together with their muscles, would then have become reduced through disuse, as would the teeth, through the not well understood principles of correlation and the economy of growth; for we everywhere see that parts which are no longer of service are reduced in size."—"*Descent of Man.*"

quently prove erroneous, is strikingly shown in these observations on the use of the cuspidatus. The simple and obvious use of this tooth, in the human species, is to tear such portions of food as are too hard or tough to be divided by the incisors; and we frequently find it far more developed in animals which are known to be exclusively frugivorous. Not only is its structure wholly unadapted for such an object as that assigned to it in the text, but there is no analogous or other ground for supposing that man was originally constructed for the pursuit and capture of living prey. His naturally erect position and the structure of the mouth would render this impossible by the means inferred by Hunter; and the possession of so perfect an instrument as the hand obviates the necessity of his ever employing any other organ for the purpose of seizing or holding food of whatever description."

Prof. William Youatt says ("The Horse," p. 226):

"At the age now under consideration (the fourth year) the tushes are almost peculiar to the horse, and castration does not appear to prevent or retard their development. All mares, however, have the germs of them in the chambers of the jaws, and they appear externally in the majority of old mares. Their use is not evident. Perhaps in the wild state of the horse they are weapons of offense, and he is enabled by them to more firmly seize and more deeply wound his enemy."\*

\* Prof. C. S. Tomes says: "In the domestic races the tusks of boars are much smaller than in the wild animal, and it is a curious fact that in domestic races which have become wild, the tusks increase in size at the same time that the bristles become more pronounced. Mr. Darwin suggests that the renewed

Surgeon J. H. Winter, the author of a work entitled "On the Horse," says:

"It is difficult to assign their use. Their position precludes the possibility of their being used as weapons of offense or defense. They may be viewed as a link of uniformity so commonly traced in the animated world."

Prof. William Percivall says that the cutting of the tushes causes the constitution more derangement than all the other teeth, and Prof. Youatt and other high authorities entertain similar views. The present chapter, therefore, is a proper one in which to discuss "the effects of dentition on the system generally." The discussion of the subject is left to well-known men. Messrs. Youatt and Percivall were many years ago the editors of "The Veterinarian," but their books are probably the best monuments to their memory. Prof. William Williams is the President of the Edinburgh Veterinary College. Prof. Youatt says ("The Horse," p. 230):

"This is the proper place to speak of the effect of dentition on the system generally. Horsemen in general think too lightly of it, and they scarcely dream of the animal suffering to any considerable degree, or growth of the teeth may perhaps be accounted for on the principle of correlation of growth, external agencies acting on the skin, and so indirectly influencing the teeth."

A strictly analogous result might or might not follow in the case of the horse. If so, the tushes would probably be used as weapons of offense and defense. It is reasonable to suppose that they were so used by the early progenitors of the horse, whose large tushes are described in the succeeding chapter by Prof. Marsh.

absolute illness being produced. Yet he who has to do with young horses will occasionally discover a considerable degree of febrile affection which he can refer to this cause alone. Fever, cough, catarrhal and cutaneous affections, diseases of the eyes, diarrhea, dysentery, loss of appetite, and general derangement will frequently be traced to irritation from teething. It is a rule scarcely admitting of the slightest deviation, that, when young horses are laboring under febrile affection, the mouth should be examined, and if the tushes are prominent and pushing against the gums, a crucial incision should be made over them."*

Prof. Percivall says ("Hippopathology," vol. ii, p. 225):

"There was a time when I treated the subject of dentition so lightly as to think that horses never suffered from such a cause. Experience, however, has altered my opinion. I now frequently discover young horses with disorders or febrile irritations the production of which I hesitate not to ascribe to teething. Many years ago I was consulted concerning a horse which had fed sparingly for a fortnight and lost rapidly in condition. His owner, a veterinary surgeon, was apprehensive about his life. Another surgeon was of opinion that the 'cudding' arose from preternatural

---

* Prof. Youatt's real sentiments are doubtless here expressed, but, unfortunately for his consistency, on page 227 of the same work, in speaking of the derangement caused by teething in children and dogs, he says: "The horse appears to feel little inconvenience. The gums and palate are occasionally somewhat hot and swollen, but the slightest scarification will remove this." Perhaps Prof. Youatt, like Prof. Percivall, changed his opinion late in life, and neglected to remove the blemish from his book.

bluntness of the molar teeth, which were filed. It was after this that I saw the horse, and I must confess I was at first quite as much at a loss to offer a satisfactory interpretation of the case as others had been. While meditating, however, after my inspection of the horse, on the apparently extraordinary nature of the case, it struck me that I had not seen the tushes. I went back into the stable and discovered two little tumors, red and hard, in the situation of the inferior tusks, which, when pressed, gave the animal insufferable pain. I instantly took out my pocket-knife and made crucial incisions through them both, from which moment the horse recovered his appetite, and by degrees his wonted condition. This case was the turning point in my practice, and caused me to look more closely into dentition.

"The cutting of the tushes, which may be likened to the eye-teeth of children, costs the constitution more derangement than all the other teeth put together; on which account, no doubt, it is that the period from the fourth to the fifth year proves so critical to the horse. Any disease, pulmonary in particular, setting in at this period, is doubly dangerous. In fact, teething is one cause of the fatality among young horses at this period.

"D'Arboval tells us to observe how the vital energy becomes augmented about the head, and upon the mucous surfaces in particular. He says: 'A local fever originates in the alveolar cavities. The gums become stretched from the pressure of the teeth against them. They dilate, sometimes split, and are red, hot, and painful. The roots compress the dental nerves and irritate the periosteal linings of the alveolar cavities. These causes will enable us to explain many morbid phenomena in horses about this, the most critical period of their lives.'

"When young horses are brought to me now for treatment," continues Prof. Percivall, "I invariably examine the teeth. Should the tusks be pushing against the gums, I let them through by incisions over their summits, and I extract any of the temporary teeth that appear to be obstructing the growth of the permanent. In this way I feel assured I have seen catarrhal and bronchial inflammations abated, coughs relieved, lymphatic and other glandular tumors about the head reduced, cutaneous eruptions got rid of, deranged bowels and urinary organs restored, appetite returned, and lost condition repaired.

"I am quite sure too little attention has been paid to the teeth in the treatment of young horses, and I would counsel those who have such charges by no means to disregard this remark, trifling as it may appear. The pathognomonic symptoms calling our attention, whether in young or old horses, if not to the teeth themselves, to the mouth in general, are large discharges of saliva from the mouth, with occasional slobbering; cudding of the food; difficulty of mastication or deglutition, or both, and stench of buccal secretion, perhaps of the breath as well."

Prof. Percivall continues the discussion of the subject of dentition and its effect on the health of the horse, dwelling more particularly on the disorder known as *lampas*. He says:

"There is connected with dentition another peculiarity in the horse which we must not allow to pass unnoticed. Although the period of teething, properly speaking, may be said to terminate at the fifth year, yet we must recollect it has been satisfactorily demonstrated that there is a process of growth going on in the teeth throughout the remainder of life; so that, in fact, at no period may the animal be said to be free from the influence of dentition. This accounts for lampas occurring in old as well as young horses, and furnishes my mind with strong proof that the tumidity of the bars of the mouth is dependent on operations going on in the teeth, and on that cause alone.

"What we nowadays understand by lampas is an unnatural prominence or tumidity of the cartilaginous bars forming the roof of the mouth. Naturally, the bars are pale-colored, whereas in a mouth affected with lampas they become red and tumid, losing their circumflecture, and swelling to a level with the crowns of the incisor teeth, and in some cases even beyond them. This apparent augmentation of substance is ascribable to congestion of blood-vessels, but not to that alone. I believe that in many cases there will be found to be some serous and albuminous infiltration into the cellular membrane attaching the bars to the hard palate, and that this will account for the length of time the swelling sometimes continues, as well as for the little relief, in regard to their diminution, which in such cases attends lancing of the gums.

"Although in young horses it is, I believe, admitted that lampas is caused by the cutting of the teeth, yet in old horses there are those who ascribe its production to other causes, and imagine it has a great deal to do with a horse's health, or rather with his feeding. That lampas may in some cases be the cause of tenderness in mastication, I do not deny; but, at the same time, I think I may safely affirm that in nine cases out of ten the cause of loss of appetite will be found elsewhere. The reason why lampas appears in aged horses is, in my opinion, as before stated, on account of the continuance of the process of growth in the teeth throughout life, with the nature and laws of which we are, in our present state of knowledge, too little acquainted to pretend to say why it should exist in one horse and not in another, or why it should only at times appear in the same horse.

"Is lampas a disease? The complaints which daily reach our ears persuade us it is. Every groom having an unthriving horse, or one that does not feed, is sure to search for lampas. If he finds it, in his mind the cause of lack of thrift is detected, and the remedy obvious—burning. Many a horse has been subjected to this torturing operation, and has thereby got added to his other ailments a foul, sloughy, carious sore on the roof of his mouth.

"Supposing that lampas be owing to the teeth, do not the teeth require removal, and not the bars of the mouth? In cutting or burning away lampas we mistake the effect for the cause. If lampas is not produced by the irritation of teething, then I would like to be informed what does cause it."

Prof. Youatt says of lampas ("The Horse," p. 219):

"It may arise from inflammation of the gums, propagated to the bars when the colt is shedding his teeth—young horses being more subject to it than others—or from some febrile tendency in the constitution generally, as when a young horse has lately been taken from grass, and has been over-fed or insufficiently exercised. It is well to examine the grinders, and more particularly the tushes, in order to ascertain whether they are making their way through the gums. If so, incisions should be made across the swollen gums, and immediate relief will follow. At times it appears in aged horses, the process of growth in the teeth of the horse continuing during life.

"The brutal custom of farriers, who sear and burn the bars with a red hot iron, is most objectionable. It is torturing the horse to no purpose, and may do serious injury. In a majority of cases the swelling will subside without medical treatment. A few mashes and gentle alteratives will give relief, but sometimes slight incisions across the bars with a lancet or penknife may be necessary. Indeed, scarification of the bars in lampas will seldom do harm, though it is not as necessary as is generally supposed."

Concerning "Diseases occurring during Dentition" Prof. William Williams says ("Principles and Practice of Veterinary Surgery," p. 476):

"In the horse the temporary grinders are replaced by permanent ones when he is from three to four years old, and in the ox at from two years and six months to two years and nine months. In cattle the cutting of the permanent molars is occasionally a matter of some difficulty owing to the unshed crowns of the temporary teeth becoming entangled with the new teeth, and thus proving a source of irritation and preventing the animal from feeding. In some parts of the country such animals are called 'rotten,' from their emaciated condition, and perhaps from the fetor emanating from the mouth. When cattle of this age stop feeding, lose condition, or drivel from the mouth, the teeth should be examined, and if the unshed molars are causing irritation, they should be removed with the forceps. Hundreds of young cattle have been sacrificed from this cause—actually dying of starvation. In the horse the same condition of the grinders may exist, but it is very unusual. The corner incisors, however, may present the same anomalous condition. Horses from four years to four years and six months old should have their teeth examined occasionally to see if all is going on well.

"Horses at four years old are subject to a distressing cough. At this age the third temporary grinder is replaced by its permanent successor, and at the same time the sixth grinder is being cut. Some irritation exists in the gums during the eruption of all the teeth, and in some instances it is excessive, extending from the gums to the fauces and larynx. This is particularly the case with the sixth grinder, and as a result of the extension of the irritation, cough is excited, usually in the morning, when the animal begins to feed. It is loud, sonorous, and prolonged, the horse frequently coughing twenty, thirty, or even forty times without ceasing. It is a throat cough, originating in laryngeal irritation.

"The treatment for this, which may be truly said to be a tooth-cough, is careful dieting on crushed food; hay, not much bran; grass, if in season, or roots if grass is not obtainable; alkaline medicines, more particularly the bicarbonate of soda; gentle aperients occasionally, if the bowels be irregular. If the fæces are fetid the fetor will be much diminished by a few doses of the hyposulphite of soda, the mouth to be gargled with some cooling mixture, such as the borate of soda or alum."

Of "Dentition Fever" Prof. Williams says ("Principles and Practice of Veterinary Surgery," p. 479):

"Horses from three to four years old are more subject to this species of dental irritation than those of a more tender age, and it is well known among horsemen that they will stand more fatigue at a more tender age than they will at this. The reason is because teething is now at the hight of its activity. When the animal is three years old, eight permanent grinders are being cut, and four permanent incisors are in active growth within the jaws. At four years of age the same number of grinders are out, and the same number of incisors are at a more advanced stage of growth within the jaws, in addition to the canine teeth, which make their appearance about this time.

"No wonder then that the eruption of so many teeth is a source of irritation and fever. The best treatment is to throw the animal off work, turn him to grass if the weather permits, or into a loose box in a well ventilated spot, and give him rest until the process of dentition is completed. If the gums are red and swollen, lancing them will prove a source of great relief."

On page 503 Prof. Williams, in speaking of cribbiting and wind-sucking, says: "Want of work and the irritation of teething are generally the causes of these vices."

# CHAPTER V.

### THE REMNANT TEETH.

*Usually regarded as Phenomenons.—The Name.—Traced to the Fossil Horses, in which (in the Pliocene Period) they "Ceased to be Functionally Developed."—Nature's Metamorphoses.—"The Agencies which are at work in Modeling Animal and Vegetable Forms."—Why Remnant Teeth are often, as it were, Prematurely Lost.—Fossil Horses and a Fossil Toothed-Bird.*

THE Remnant or "so-called wolf-teeth" are one of the most interesting features of the horse's dental system. They are generally regarded as phenomenons, but their line of descent is as direct as that of the first premolars (grinders), which have, as it were, almost absorbed them, and have increased in bulk nearly in proportion to the decrease in bulk of the Remnant teeth.

As the word "wolf" is another name for that which is hurtful or destructive, and as these teeth as well as supernumerary teeth, with which, however, they should never be confounded, sometimes do injury, the generic name, "wolf-teeth," is not a bad one. But, since these particular teeth are hereditary, being beyond doubt the remains of teeth that were once functionally developed, they require a specific name; I have therefore adopted the name REMNANT TEETH.

In the evolution of the horse from an animal of about the size of a fox to his present proportions, it is not strange that radical physical changes, of the teeth as well as other organs, should have occurred, or that they are in harmony with his bodily requirements as well as his usefulness to man. Small, four-toed limbs would support the body of an animal no larger than a fox or a sheep, but they would require additional size and strength to support the small horse (Hipparion) of the Pliocene period, or the large horse of the present period (Equus). This additional strength was gradually acquired by the enlargement of the limbs and the solidification, as it were, of four toes into one, it being as natural, in conformity to the law of adaptation, for a line of succeeding animal forms to undergo bodily changes as for an individual form to do so.

During these metamorphoses equally varied and interesting changes occurred in the horse's dental system, which are described by Prof. O. C. Marsh, of Yale College, in the article "Horse, Fossil," in "Johnson's New Universal Cyclopedia (vol. ii, p. 996). He gives a general description of the changes that have occurred in species of three geological periods, namely, the Pliocene, Miocene, and Eocene, those of the two last named having forty-four functionally developed teeth. The part of the article which refers to the teeth is as follows:

"In the Pliocene tertiary period the horse was represented by several extinct genera, the best known being Hipparion (or Hippotherium). The species are small, as the name implies, Hipparion being a diminutive from the Greek *hippos*, a 'horse.' In the upper molar teeth there is in Hipparion, on the anterior portion of the inner side, an isolated ellipse of enamel inclosing dentine, and not joined with the main body of the tooth by an isthmus of dentine, as in *Equus*, at least until the teeth are nearly worn out. Anchippus, also from the Pliocene, resembled in its teeth Anchitherium of the Miocene, a genus now considered as typical of a family distinct from that of the horse. In Anchitherium the molars have short crowns, devoid of cement, and are inserted by distinct roots. The Miocene species were not larger than a sheep. The Eocene representatives of the group were still smaller, the largest hardly exceeding a fox in size. They belong to the genus Orohippus. The dentition is very similar to that of Anchitherium, but the first upper premolar is larger and the succeeding ones smaller than in that genus. The diastema, or 'place for the bit,' is distinct. The canines are large, and near the incisors. The crowns of the molars are short and destitute of cement, and the skeleton is decidedly equine in its general features.

"'The gradual elongation of the head and neck may be said to have already begun in Orohippus, if we compare that form with other most nearly allied mammals. The diastema was well developed even then, but increased materially in succeeding genera. The number of teeth remained the same until the Pliocene, when the *front lower premolar was lost, and subsequently the corresponding upper tooth ceased to be functionally developed.*\* The next upper premolar, which in Orohippus was the smallest of the six posterior

---

\* The italics are mine. This "corresponding upper tooth that ceased to be functionally developed," is the identical tooth that now appears as a mere remnant.

teeth, rapidly increased in size, and finally became the largest of the series. The grinding teeth had at first very short crowns, without cement, and were inserted by distinct roots. In Pliocene species the molars became longer, and were more or less coated with cement. The modern horse has very long grinders, without true roots, which are covered with a thick external layer of cement. The large canines of Orohippus became gradually reduced in the later genera, and the characteristic 'mark' upon the incisors is found only in the later forms. It is an interesting fact that the peculiarly equine features acquired by Orohippus are retained persistently throughout the entire series of succeeding forms."*

* "The ancient Orohippus had all four digits of the fore-feet well developed. In Mesohippus, of the next period, the fifth toe is only represented by a rudiment, and the limb is supported by the second, third, and fourth, the middle one being the largest. Hipparion of the Later Tertiary still has three digits, but the third is much stouter, and the outer toes have ceased to be of use, as they do not touch the ground. In Equus the lateral hoofs are gone, and the digits themselves are represented only by the rudimentary splint-bones. The middle or third digit supports the limb, and its size has increased accordingly. The corresponding changes in the posterior limb of these genera are very similar but not so striking, as the oldest type (Orohippus) had but three toes behind. The earlier ancestor of the group, perhaps in the lowest Eocene, probably had four on this foot and five in front. Such a predecessor is as clearly indicated by the feet of Orohippus as the latter is by its Miocene relative. A still older ancestor, possibly in the Cretaceous, doubtless had five toes on each foot, the typical number in mammals. This reduction in the number of toes may perhaps have been due to elevation of the region inhabited, which gradually led the animals to live on higher ground, instead of the soft lowlands, where a many-toed foot would be most useful."—*Prof. O. C. Marsh.*

The article closes as follows:

"Such is, in brief, a general outline of the more marked changes that appear to have produced in America the highly specialized modern Equus from its diminutive, four-toed predecessor, the Eocene Orohippus. The line of descent appears to have been direct, and the remains now known supply every important intermediate form. Considering the remarkable development of the group throughout the entire tertiary period, and its existence even later, it seems very strange that none of the species should have survived, and that we are indebted for our present horse to the Old World."*

* The following extracts from Prof. C. S. Tomes's "Dental Anatomy, Human and Comparative" (pp. 247-8, 254-5), explain some of the causes of the metamorphoses described by Prof. Marsh: "He would indeed be a rash man who ventured to assert that we had recognized all the agencies which are at work in the modeling of animal and vegetable forms; but it is safe to say that, at the present time, we are acquainted with several agencies which are in constant operation, and which are competent to profoundly modify animals in successive generations. We know of 'natural selection,' or 'survival of the fittest,' an agency by which variations beneficial to their possessors will be preserved and intensified in successive generations; of 'sexual selection,' which operates principally by enabling those possessed of certain characters to propagate their race, while others less favored do not get the opportunity of so doing; of 'concomitant variation' between different parts of the body, an agency much more recondite in its operations, but by which agencies affecting one part may secondarily bring about alterations in some other part.

"The doctrine of natural selection, or survival of the fittest, is as applicable to the teeth of an animal as to any part of its organization, and the operation of this natural law will be constantly tending to produce advantages or 'adaptive' differences. On the other hand, the strong power of inheritance is tending to

## NOT RARE, BUT EASILY LOST. 99

Remnant teeth are not rare, but it is rare for them to persist in the jaws till even middle age. However, preserve even that which, in the altering conditions of life, has become of very little use. Thus we may understand rudimentary teeth to be teeth which are in process of disappearance, having ceased to be useful to their possessors, but still for a time, through the influence of inheritance, lingering upon the scene. Some teeth have disappeared utterly. Thus the upper incisors of ruminants are gone, and no rudiments exist at any stage; others still remain in a stunted form, and do not persist throughout the lifetime of the animal, as, for instance, the first premolars of the horse, or two out of the four premolars of most bears.

"Teeth are profoundly susceptible of modification, but amid all their varied forms, the evidences of descent from ancestors whose teeth departed less from the typical mammalian dentition are clearly traceable by the existence of rudimentary teeth and other such characters. * * * The power of inheritance is constantly asserting itself by the retention, for a time at least, of parts which have become useless, and by the occasional reappearance of characters which have been lost. * * * Things that are rudimentary often teach us most; for being of no present use, they are not undergoing that rapid change in adaptation to the animal's habits which may be going on in organs that are actively employed."

Horses are not the only animals that have had or are having changes in their dentition. Mr. C. R. Darwin says ("Descent of Man," vol. i, p. 25): "It appears as if the posterior molar or wisdom-teeth were tending to become rudimentary in the more civilized races of men. They are rather smaller than the other teeth. In the Melanian races, on the other hand, the wisdom-teeth are usually furnished with three separate fangs, are generally sound, and differ in size from the other molars less than in the Caucasian races. Prof. Schaaffhausen accounts for this difference between the races by 'the posterior dental portion of the jaw being always shortened' in those that are civilized, and this shortening may, I presume, be safely attributed to civilized men habitually feeding on soft, cooked food, and thus using their jaws less. I am informed by Mr. Brace that it is becoming quite a common practice in the United States to remove some

there may be cases where they never appear; but it by no means follows that because a horse is not in possession of them that he never had any. There are various causes for their frequent absence, but the chief cause is their small size. Remnant teeth of the lower jaw, which are very rare, are probably cases of "reversion to a former state."* If these latter teeth were not expelled in the manner explained below by Mons.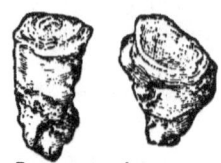
Remnant teeth; natural size.—*Original*.
Lecoq, the probability is that they would not long withstand the friction of the bit. The upper teeth, however, while they may sometimes be expelled by the bit, are comparatively little disturbed by it, which probably accounts for their now and then remaining in the jaws for years. Another reason for their persistence is that their roots are long in proportion to their bodies. The reason why these teeth should not be confounded with supernumerary or abnormal teeth will appear in the succeeding chapter, which is devoted to the consideration of the latter.

Monsieur Lecoq gives cogent reasons for the frequent absence of Remnant teeth. He says:

"Supplementary molars are sometimes met with in front of the true ones, and there may be four of them, two in either jaw, above and below. They are small teeth, having but little resemblance to the others, are frequently shed with the first deciduous molar, and are not replaced. The first replacing (permanent) molar is always a little more elongated than that of the molar teeth of children, as the jaw does not grow large enough for the perfect development of the normal number."

\* See the second reference note, page 80.

which it succeeds, and it frequently expels at the same time the supplementary molar; so that if forty-four teeth be developed in the male horse, it is very rare that they are all present at the same time."

That Remnant teeth are usually regarded as phenomenons is abundantly proved by some of the extracts that follow. In "Johnson's New Universal Cyclopedia" (p. 995), article "Horse," it is said:

"An additional small tooth is occasionally found in advance of the upper molar series. This tooth, when present, is the smallest of all the teeth, and, as it has neither predecessor nor successor, its nature is in doubt."

As the nature of these teeth appeared to be clearly explained in the article "Horse, Fossil," which immediately follows that on the "Horse," I wrote to Prof. Joseph Leidy, telling him I believed the "wolf-teeth" were the remnants of the teeth that "ceased to be functionally developed," and asked his opinion about the matter. Writing under date of "Philadelphia, Nov. 26, 1878," he said:

\* \* \* "I think you are right in supposing that the little premolars referred to by Prof. Marsh as the 'corresponding upper teeth,' which 'ceased to be functionally developed,' are the so-called 'wolf-teeth.'"

Another letter, addressed to Prof. Theodore Gill, elicited the following reply, which was dated "Smithsonian Institution, Washington, D. C., Nov. 25. 1878:"

\* \* \* "The complete dentition of the adult horse is represented by the formula: I., $\frac{3}{3}$; C., $\frac{1}{1}$; D., $\frac{1}{0}$; P. M., $\frac{3}{3}$; M., $\frac{3}{3} \times 2 = 42$. The 'small wolf or supernumerary tooth that appears in front of the first upper premolar,' is the more or less persistent first deciduous molar (d 1) of the first series, which is not succeeded by a first premolar. The premolars are consequently P. M., 2, 3, and 4 of the typical educabilian dentition."

Prof. Richard Owen, who, like Drs. Gill and Leidy, has a clear conception of the subject, says:

"The second incisor appears between the twentieth and fortieth days, and about this time the first small, deciduous premolar takes its place. * * * The representative of the first premolar is a very small and simple rudiment, and is soon shed."

Surgeon Charles Parnell, in a letter to the editor of "The Veterinarian" (1867, p. 287), says:

"In reading Prof. George Varnell's articles on some of the diseases affecting the facial region of the horse's head, I notice a description of wolf-teeth. He says: 'They have been supposed to be the cause of disease in the eyes of horses. This idea, however, is quite erroneous; therefore I shall not occupy any space in discussing this traditional error.' Well, I can safely say that I have in my time extracted a great many of these teeth, and not merely because they existed, but because there was a weeping from both eyes, the cause of which was attributed to wolf-teeth, and generally in the course of a few weeks the weeping has ceased. But what convinces me that they do affect the eye is that in several cases where there were weeping and weakness of one eye only, I have found a wolf-tooth on the affected side only, and the recovery of the eye has invariably followed the extraction of the tooth. The mucous membranes and lachrymal glands appear to be the parts affected, undoubtedly from some connection through the nerves. If these teeth are allowed to remain in the horse's mouth, the sight will become more or less impaired."

Might not this plan (extracting the teeth), if adopted by all surgeons, eventually rid horses of the so-called wolf-teeth? Nature may be aided or injured. The effect of interfering with nature is illustrated by the following extract from Prof. W. Youatt's work, "The Horse" (p. 154):

"The custom of cropping the ears of the horse originated, to its shame, in Great Britain, and for many years was a practice not only cruel to the animal, but deprived it of much of its beauty. It was so obstinately persisted in that at length the deformity became in some hereditary, and a breed of horses born without ears was produced."

Extracting the Remnant teeth appears to aid rather than injure nature. The practice is therefore as commendable as the cropping of the ears is reprehensible, and if the same result should follow that Prof. Youatt says followed the cropping of the ears, it ought to be adopted.

C. D. House, an American veterinary dentist, like Surgeon Parnell, invariably extracts the Remnant teeth. He not only claims that they sometimes injure the eyes, but that in some cases, when they encroach on the maxillary branch of the fifth pair of nerves, they cause the horse to act as if insane. He says he has more than once extracted these teeth when the "insane" horse was in an open field. When the tooth is drawn and the animal is relieved, it looks around and stares and acts as if wondering where it is and how it got there. Not more than one horse in twenty possessing these teeth, he says, ever suffers injury to its eyes.

Surgeon R. Jennings of Detroit has examined many fetuses and always found Remnant teeth germs; during 37 years' practice, in more than 100 deaths under two years, not a single instance occurred where these teeth, or the germs which produce them, were not found. They will be found usually at the age of two years.

Veterinary Dentist J. Ramsey of Boston treated a 7-year-old horse in 1881 that had been "out of condition" for several years, and consequently had had *several* owners. He discovered a long Remnant tooth with such a vicious inclination toward the roof of the mouth as to interfere with the use of the tongue. As soon as the tooth was extracted the horse began to eat.

Prof. Williams says of Remnant teeth ("Principles and Practice of Veterinary Surgery," p. 479):

"Small supernumerary teeth are often met with in front of the grinders, called 'wolf-teeth.' They have been supposed to be a cause of ophthalmia, but this is doubtful. They can produce no inconvenience; but if requested to extract them a practitioner can hardly refuse. The best method is to remove them with the tooth-forceps.

"The question as to the influence of the teeth on the eyes might perhaps be deemed worthy of discussion, inasmuch as the dental nerve is a branch of that which supplies the eyes with common sensibility, namely, the fifth. The older writers maintained that 'moon-blindness' was due to wolf-teeth, and the first procedure in the treatment was their removal. Nowadays, however, the supposition is not carried quite so far, and the utmost that can be said is that the irritation of teething may be an exciting cause of ophthalmia in animals whose constitutions are hereditarily or otherwise predisposed to the disease, and the removal of supernumerary teeth, or lancing the gums, may possibly be followed by some remission of the ophthalmic symptoms."

Prof. Youatt thus accounts for Remnant teeth:

"In a few instances the permanent teeth do not rise immediately under the temporary, but somewhat by their side. Then, instead of the gradual process of absorption, the root, being compressed sideways, diminishes throughout its whole bulk. The crown diminishes also, and the tooth is pushed out of its place to the forepart of the first grinder, and remains for a considerable time under the name of a *wolf-tooth*, causing swelling and soreness of the gums, and frequently wounding the cheeks. They would be gradually quite absorbed, but the process might be slow and the annoyance great; therefore they are extracted."

Prof. Youatt's theory is unique, but it fails to give a satisfactory explanation of the "so-called wolf-teeth." That a tooth should be pushed out of its place is simple enough; but why would the first upper temporary grinder remain in the gum and take root and the first lower not? That "they would be gradually quite absorbed," is disproved by the fact that they sometimes persist till old age; and this fact also disproves the assertion that "they are extracted." Some surgeons do not extract them. Prof. Youatt doubtless meant to say they *should* be extracted.

As Remnant teeth are found functionally developed in the jaws of fossil horses—in which they were the largest of all the teeth—a few extracts from the works of well-known men concerning fossil horses and their teeth will be appropriate as a conclusion to this chapter. Prof. Richard Owen says ("Odontography," vol. i, p. 575):

"Cuvier was unable, from the materials at his command, to detect any characters in the bones or teeth of the different existing species of *Equus*, or in the fossil remains of the same genus, by which he could distinguish them, save by their difference of size. Among the numerous teeth of a species of *Equus* as large as a horse fourteen and a half hands high, collected from the Oreston cavernous fissures, I have found specimens clearly indicating two distinct species, so far as specific differences may be founded on well-marked modifications of the teeth.

"One of these, like the ordinary *Equus fossilis* of the drift and pleistocene formations, differs from the existing *Equus caballus* by the minor transverse diameter of the molar teeth; the other, in the more complex and elegant plication of the enamel,* and in the

---

\* In Prof. Owen's "History of British Fossil Mammals and Birds" (pp. 393-4), the "elegant plication of the enamel" on the crown of this tooth is illustrated. Prof. Owen says: "Fig. 153 illustrates the character, above adverted to, of the complex plication of the enamel, as it appears on the grinding surface of a partially worn upper molar tooth, the second of the right side. The length of this tooth is three inches four lines, and the fangs had not begun to be formed. One cannot view the elegant foldings of the enamel in the present fossil teeth, and in those of

bilobed posterior termination of the grinding surface of the last upper molar, more closely approximates to the extinct horse of the Miocene period, which Herr von Meyer has characterized under the name of *Equus caballus primigenius*. The Oreston fossil teeth differ, however, from this in the form of the fifth or internal prism of dentine in the upper molars, and in its continuation with the anterior lobe of the teeth, the fifth prism being oval and insulated in the *Equus primigenius* of Von Meyer.

"The Oreston fossil teeth, which in their principal characters manifest so close a relationship with the Miocene *Equus primigenius*, differ, like the later drift species (*Eq. fossilis*), from the recent horse in a greater proportional antero-posterior diameter of the crown, and also in a less produced anterior angle of the first premolar. I have named this British fossil horse *Equus plicidens*. The fossil horse (*Eq. curvidens*) of South America, which coexisted with the megatherium,† and, like it, became extinct apparently before

---

the more ancient primigenial species (Hippotheria) of the continental Miocene deposits, without being reminded of the peculiar character of the enamel of the molars of the Elasmotherium, in which it is folded in elegant festoons. This extinct pachyderm, which surpassed the rhinoceros in size, resembled that genus very closely in the general disposition of the folds of enamel in the grinding teeth, but agreed with the modern horse in the deep implantation of those teeth by an undivided base. The Elasmothere appears, therefore, to have formed one of the links, now lost, which connected the horse with the rhinoceros; and it is interesting to observe that some of the extinct species of horse, in the analogous complexity of the enamel folds, more closely resembled the Elasmothere than do the present species."

† "The teeth of this most gigantic of the extinct quadrupeds of the sloth tribe are small in proportion to the size of the ani-

the introduction of the human race, differs from the existing horse by the greater degree of curvature of the upper molars."

The following account of two fossil molar teeth of an extinct species of horse, discovered in South America, may be found in Prof. Owen's "Fossil Mammalia and Mammalia," (pp. 108–9):

"*Notice of the remains of a species of Equus, found associated with the extinct Edentals and Toxodon at Punta Alta, in Bahia Blanca, and with the Mastodon and Toxodon at Santa Fé, in Entre Rios.*—The first of these remains is a superior molar tooth of the right side. It was imbedded in the quartz shingle, formed of pebbles strongly cemented together with calcareous matter, which adhered as closely to it as the corresponding matrix did to the associated fossil remains. The tooth was as completely fossilized as the remains of the mylodon, megatherium, and scelidothere, and was so far decomposed that in the attempt to detach the adherent matrix it became partially resolved into its component curved lamellæ. Every point of comparison that could be established proved it to differ from the tooth of the common *Equus caballus* only in a slight inferiority of size.

"The second evidence of the coexistence of the horse with the extinct mammals of the tertiary epoch of South America reposes on a more perfect tooth, likewise of the upper jaw, from the red argillaceous

mal. They are five in number on each side of the upper jaw, and, probably, four on each side of the lower. They present a more or less tetragonal figure, and have the grinding surface traversed by two transverse angular ridges."—*Owen*.

earth of the Pampas at Bojada de Santa Fé, in the Province of Entre Rios. This tooth agreed so closely in color and condition with the remains of the mastodon and toxodon, from the same locality, that I have no doubt respecting the contemporaneous existence of the individual horse of which it once formed part. This tooth is figured at Plate xxxii, Figs. 13 and 14, from which the anatomist can judge of its close correspondence with a middle molar of the left side of the upper jaw.

"This evidence of the former existence of a genus which, as regards South America, had become extinct, and has a second time been introduced into that continent, is not one of the least interesting points of Mr. Darwin's paleontological discoveries." *

---

* Mr. Darwin, in his work on "The Descent of Man" (vol. i, pp. 230-1), says: "Although the gradual decrease and final extinction of the races of man is an obscure problem, we can see that it depends on many causes, differing in different places and at different times. It is the same difficult problem as that presented by the extinction of one of the higher animals—of the fossil horse, for instance—which disappeared from South America, soon to be replaced, within the same districts, by countless herds of the Spanish horse."

In his "Journal of Researches" (pp. 130-1-2), Mr. Darwin gives further information concerning the fossil teeth described by Prof. Owen, and advances a theory of the introduction of the horse into the "so-called New World." He says: "In the Pampæan deposit of the Bojada I found the osseous armor of a gigantic, armadillo-like animal, the inside of which, when the earth was removed, was like a great cauldron. I also found teeth of the toxodon and mastodon, and one of a horse, in the same stained and decayed state. The latter greatly interested me, and I took scrupulous care in ascertaining that it had been imbedded contemporaneously with the other remains; for I was not then aware that among the fossils from Bahia Blanca there

Prof. Thomas H. Huxley says ("Critiques and Addresses," pp. 191-5):

"Let us endeavor to find some cases of true linear types, or forms which are intermediate between others, because they stand in a direct genetic relation to them. It is no easy matter to find clear and unmistakable evidence of filiation among fossil animals. After much

was a horse's tooth hidden in the matrix; nor was it then known with certainty that the remains of horses were common in North America. Mr. Lyell has lately brought from the United States a tooth of a horse; and it is an interesting fact that Prof. Owen could find in no species, either fossil or recent, a slight but peculiar curvature characterizing it, until he thought of comparing it with my specimen found here. Certainly it is a marvelous fact in the history of the Mammalia, that in South America a native horse should have lived and disappeared, to be succeeded in after ages by the countless herds descended from the few introduced by the Spanish colonists! (1 need hardly state here that there is good evidence against any horse living in America at the time of Columbus).

"When America, and especially North America, possessed its elephants, mastodons, horse, and hollow-horned ruminants, it was much more closely related in its zoölogical characters to the temperate parts of Europe and Asia than it now is. As the remains of these genera are found on both sides of Behring's Straits and on the plains of Siberia, we are led to look to the northwestern side of North America as the former point of communication between the Old and the so called New World. And as so many species, both living and extinct, of these same genera inhabit and have inhabited the Old World, it seems most probable that the North American elephants, mastodons, horse, and hollow-horned ruminants migrated—on land since submerged near Behring's Straits—from Siberia into North America, and thence—on land since submerged in the West Indies—into South America, where for a time they mingled with the forms characteristic of that southern continent, and have since become extinct."

search, however, I think that such a case is to be made out in favor of the horses. The modern horse is represented as far back as the latter part of the Miocene epoch; but in deposits belonging to the middle of that epoch its place is taken by two other genera, Hipparion and Anchitherium. A species of Anchitherium was referred by Cuvier to the Paleotheria. The grinding teeth are in fact very similar in shape and in pattern, and in the absence of any thick layer of cement, to those of some species of Paleotherium. But in the fact that there are only six full-sized grinders in the lower jaw, the first premolar being very small; that the anterior grinders are as large as or rather larger than the posterior ones; that the second premolar has an anterior prolongation, and that the posterior molar of the lower jaw has, as Cuvier pointed out, a posterior lobe of much smaller size and different form, the dentition of Anchitherium departs from the type of the Paleotherium and approaches that of the horse. The skeleton of Anchitherium is extremely equine.

"In the Hipparion the teeth nearly resemble those of the horse, though the crowns of the grinders are not so long. Like those of the horse, they are abundantly coated with cement. In the modern horse, finally, the crowns of the grinding teeth become longer, and their patterns are slightly modified."

Alfred Russel Wallace, F.R.G.S., &c., says ("The Geographical Distribution of Animals," New York edition, vol. i, p. 135):

"*Ungulata.*—The animals belonging to this order being usually of large size and accustomed to feed and travel in herds, are liable to wholesale destruction by floods, bogs, precipices, drought, or hunger. It is for these reasons, probably, that their remains are almost always more numerous than those of other orders of mammalia. In America they are especially abundant.

"The true horses are represented in the Pliocene by several ancestral forms. The most nearly allied to the modern horse is Pliohippus, consisting of animals about the size of an ass, with lateral toes not externally developed, but with some differences of dentition. Next come Protohippus and Hipparion, in which the lateral toes are developed, but are small and functionless, Protohippus being only two feet and a half high. Then we have the allied genera, Anchippus, Merychippus, and Hyohippus, which were still smaller animals. In the older deposits we come to a series of forms, still unmistakably equine, but with three or more toes used for locomotion, and with numerous differentiations in form, proportions, and dentition. In the Miocene we have the genera Anchitherium, Miohippus, and Mesohippus, with three toes on each foot, and about the size of a sheep or large goat. In the Eocene of Utah and Wyoming we get a step further back, several species having been discovered about the size of a fox, with four toes in front and three behind. These form the genus Orohippus, and are the oldest ancestral horse known."

The following account of a horse's tooth that was found while digging a well is from *The Popular Science Review:*

"In a paper read before the St. Louis Academy of Science, and reported in *The American Naturalist* for March, 1871, Mr. G. C. Broadhead records some interesting facts about fossil horses. Alluding to the fact that horse remains have been found in the altered drift of Kansas, he says he is now able to announce that similar remains have been discovered in a well at Papinville, Bates County, Mo. Mr. O. P. Ohlinger, while digging a well, unearthed a tooth at a depth of thirty-one feet from the surface; it was resting in a bed of sand beneath a 4-inch stratum of bluish clay and gravel. Beneath the sand containing the tooth was a gravel-bed five feet in thickness. He sent the tooth to Prof. Joseph Leidy, of Philadelphia, who pronounced it to be the last upper molar of a horse, probably an extinct species."

In various volumes of the "Proceedings of the Academy of Natural Sciences of Philadelphia," accounts of many other fossil horses' teeth may be found, of which the following is a specimen ("Proceedings," &c., 1871, p. 113):

"Prof. Joseph Leidy exhibited a specimen of an upper molar tooth, which Mr. Timothy Conrad had picked up from a pile of Miocene marl at Greenville, Pitt County, N. C. He believed, from its size and the intricacy in the folding of the enamel of the islets at the middle of the triturating surface, that the tooth belonged to the Post-Pliocene *Equus complicatus*, and was an accidental occupant of the Miocene marl. It might, however, belong to a Hipparion of the Miocene period, but the imperfection of the specimen at its inner part prevented its positive generic determination."

The discoveries of horse remains since 1880 by Prof. E. D. Cope, one of the editors of *The American Naturalist*, are of an extraordinary character, and an interesting account of them appears in the APPENDIX to this work. Truly the Americas are rich in fossil remains, and it is becoming a common thing to hear of the unearthing of mastodons, elephants, etc.

NOTE.—The birds of the present epoch are entirely destitute of true teeth, and the mandibles have generally more or less trenchant, unarmed linear edges; but sometimes they are armed with processes of bone simulating teeth, but in no other respect entitled to that name. In former epochs, however, there existed types actually provided with true teeth, having all the structural characteristics of those organs, and fitting in sockets in the jaws. These have been combined by Marsh under the general term Odontornithes (toothed birds).—*Gill.*

The teeth of *Hesperornis* were covered with smooth enamel, terminating upward in conical pointed crowns and downward in stout roots. The young tooth probably formed on the inner side of the root of the tooth in use, a pit for its reception being gradually made by absorption. The old tooth, being progressively undermined, was finally expelled by its successor, the number of teeth thus remaining unchanged. The teeth were implanted in a common alveolar groove, as in *Ichthyosaurus.* The skeleton measures about 6 feet from the point of the tail to the end of the bill. *Hesperornis regalis* appears to have had 14 functional teeth in the upper and 33 in the lower jaw.—*Marsh.*

A fossil is the body or any known part or trace of an animal or plant buried by natural causes in the earth. The molds of shells, the impressions left by the feet of animals in walking, implements of stone or metal, and other works of human art which have been accumulated naturally into rubbish-heaps, are thus strictly fossils. Perhaps the marks of rain, wind, waves, and shrinkage through heat should be included. \* \* \* Fossils indicate the former existence of organic races now entirely extinct ; that, as a whole, each successive period contained more highly organized structures than its predecessor; that tropical forms once flourished in the polar regions; that each epoch was characterized by peculiar groups. Hence, formations are identified in new countries by means of fossils.— *C. H. Hitchcock.*

For interesting articles on Fossil Botany, Fossil Fishes, Fossil Footprints, and Fossil Forests, the reader is referred to Johnson's " New Universal Cyclopedia," vol. ii, pp. 231–9.

# CHAPTER VI.

### DENTAL CYSTS AND SUPERNUMERARY TEETH.

Teeth growing in various parts of the Body.—Some Cysts more Prolific than others, Producing a Second, if not a Third, "Dentition."—Reports and Theories of Scientific Men.—Cases of Third Dentition in Human Beings.

THE development of abnormal teeth in different parts of the body (the human body as well as those of the lower animals, particularly the horse), is not the least interesting feature in the study of dental science. To judge from the reports that follow, one would think the tooth-substance in some horses was an unknown quantity. It would be interesting and useful to know whether in such cases the natural teeth are in a perfectly healthy state, and whether the temperature is natural, instead of being increased, as during certain periods of teething. While the study of these teeth may not be of paramount importance, it serves to further illustrate the physiological relations of the dental system, and ought to assist the surgeon in more correctly diagnosing diseases.

Surgeon George Fleming, of the Royal Engineers, contributed a valuable paper entitled "Dental Cysts, or Tooth-Bearing Tumors," to "The Veterinarian" for 1874 (p. 692), the substance of which is as follows:

"In *The Gazetta Medico-Veterinaria* of Milan for 1873 (p. 274), Profs. Lanzillotti-Buonsanti and Guiseppe Generali, of the Veterinary School of that city, published a most complete and interesting contribution to our knowledge of the pathology of dental cysts in the horse, well illustrated with wood-cuts, and including a full bibliographical record and synoptical table of these morbid productions. From their researches it would appear that dental cysts were first described by Mage Grouillé, in 1811.*

"These teeth-bearing tumors have received different names. Thus they have been designated 'erratic' or 'misplaced teeth,' 'dental neoplasies,' 'odontocysts,' 'dental degeneration of the temporal bone,' 'temporal fistula,' 'abnormal development of teeth in unusual places,' 'auricular teeth,' 'odontocele,' and 'dentigerous cysts' or 'teeth tumors.' They may be developed in unusual places, such as the temporal region, the frontal bones, the base of the ear, the space between the branches of the lower jaw, the lumbar region, the testicles, and the ovaries. Coleman stands alone in his case of a cyst found beneath the right kidney, in which were two small molars and an incisor, attached to a bone that resembled a jaw, though the Milan professors believe the teeth in this instance may have been developed in a testicle retained in the abdominal cavity. The most common situation is undoubtedly in the temporal region, as in seventy-five recorded cases sixty-eight were observed there. These cases all refer to the horse. Berger-Perriere, however, found a temporary incisor in a fistulous wound near the right ear

---

* "No mention is made of the Αἱδοιγενομένοι ἐν τοῖς γνάδοις, or maxillary exostoses of Apsyrtus ('Hipp. Gr.' p. 64), who recommends that these tumors should be carefully and completely removed, or they will return of a larger size."

The reference note is also Surgeon Fleming's.

of a lamb two months and a half old ('Recueil de Méd. Vétérinaire,' 1835, p. 586).

"In most instances only one tooth is found. Gurlt was the first to find, on the mastoid process of the temporal bone, a mass of molar teeth fused, as it were, together. The tumor was three inches and a half high, and about two in its largest diameter. The horse had been destroyed for glanders. Goubaux found two at the posterior portion of the sphenoid bone, and Bay four. In a cyst of the testicle Gurlt discovered six teeth, three separate and three in a mass. Bay attended a horse in 1860 that appeared to be suffering with encephalitis. It died twenty-four hours after his visit. It had always shown, on the right temporal region, a tumor without a fistula, but it did not attract notice, as it apparently caused no inconvenience. Nine years afterward, when Bay was preparing the head as a pathological specimen, he discovered this supposed exostosis to be constituted by the union of four molar teeth. The two superior teeth projected from the temporal articulation, and the inferior two were situated in the petrous portion of the temporal bone, inclining obliquely from within outward. The posterior portion of the latter projected in a very salient manner at the *sella turcica*, and must have produced much pressure on important parts of the brain.

"Age does not appear to have any influence on the development of these cysts, the animals in which they have been observed ranging in age from eight or nine months to fifteen years. The period of formation also varied greatly. In regard to the side of the body in which they were developed, in seventeen cases they were on the left, and in thirteen on the right. In fourteen cases observed by Macrops, they were indifferently on both sides. In this respect clinical observation has not yielded any fact of practical importance.

"Sometimes, after the extraction of a tooth, it happens that the cavity of the cyst or the bottom of the fistula does not cicatrize. This is a sure indication that a new tooth is forming. Rodet noted this fact as long ago as 1827. Macrops has observed a case of this kind. He was compelled to operate twice within three months, each time removing a molar tooth; and when he made his report, in 1860, it was probable that a third tooth was being developed, as the fistula had not closed."

Surgeon Fleming also mentions cases that were observed by Surgeons Perosino, Martin, Harold, Gamgee, Coclet, Lafosse, and others. He continues:

"Profs. Lanzillotti-Buonsanti and Generali made minute inspection of a specimen of tooth taken from the base of the ear of a foal twenty months old, and they report that microscopically the structure of such teeth does not differ much from natural teeth. The same constituents—dentine, enamel, and cement—were found, the only difference being that they were arranged in an unusual manner. In the tooth they examined, for instance, the cement was abundant in the central part, while in that studied by Oreste and Falconio, the dentine was most abundant and the cement least in quantity."

Surgeon Fleming next refers to and gives a summary of the views of scientific men, who say that "A certain number of teeth may sometimes be developed as parasitic productions in a cavity similar to and situated near the mouth (in which category is included the excellent case occurring in a woman, and described, in 1862, by Prof. Generali—an observation unique in the teratology of mankind—namely, a case of parasitic monstrosity, in which, however, the designation 'dental cyst,' so inexact in itself, is inappropriate and false);" that "the ovarian cysts in women, in which have been found pieces of bone and cartilage, teeth, and a lower jaw, more or less deformed, ought to be considered as probable cases of ovarian impregnation with an incompletely developed fetus, and in young girls as examples of the intra-uterine formation of a fetus within a fetus;" that "only in this way can be explained the lipomatous and sarcomatous congenital masses contained in cysts, with the teeth and fragments of bone simulating an incomplete jaw, which have been observed on the human orbit (Lobstein and Travers), on the palate (Otto), on the tongue (Stansky), on the side of the jaw, in the cheek, and on the neck, but which Schultze and Panum consider as the simple proliferation of embryonic plasmatic cells;" that "some dental cysts are true dermoid cysts, containing hair and teeth," &c., and closes his paper with the following common-sense suggestion:

"Perhaps direct researches, which have not yet been made, carried out in favorable circumstances, will better serve in deciding their real nature than all the more or less brilliant academical reasoning."

John Gamgee, Professor of Anatomy and Physiology in the Edinburgh Veterinary College, in the course of a series of articles on various subjects in "The Veterinarian" for 1856, thus comments on a case of dentigerous cyst, the history of which was originally written by Monsieur Lafosse and published in the "Journal des Vétérinaire du Midi:"

"M. Lafosse, Professor of Clinical Medicine in the Veterinary School of Toulouse, had under his treatment a four-year-old mare that for two months before admission into the infirmary was affected with a phlegmonous tumor in the region of the left ear. This was opened. The wound that resulted rapidly contracted, but a fistula remained. When Lafosse first saw the case, he found a painful tumor, with a granulating wound just behind the scutiform cartilage, and near the upper part of the parotid gland. By probing he ascertained that at the bottom of the fistulous tract was some hard substance, which he supposed to be the scutiform cartilage in an ossified state, or a portion of the temporal bone exfoliating. A severe operation was performed, and the solid substance extracted. It was double, deeply seated, and firmly adherent to surrounding textures. Slight hemorrhage ensued from the division of the anterior auricular, but was easily stopped. The wound was dressed, and the animal soon recovered, having shown only a few symptoms of sore throat after the operation.

"I shall not translate M. Lafosse's description of the products he extracted. They were composed of tooth-substance, and although it has been questioned whether it is real tooth that is developed in the shape of accidental growths in the region of the ear, still the fact is now well established, however puzzling to the minds of some it may be to comprehend their origin.

"Lafosse attempts a teratological explanation, but asks: 'If teeth are looked on as arising from the tegumentary system, considering them in most animals as emanating from papillæ and mucous membrane, where was the dermoid papilla that constituted the basis of development of this tooth, deeply seated and close to the ear, especially as what might be taken as the crown looked toward the inner surface of the skin?'

"Further on Lafosse shows that in certain animals teeth absolutely emanate from the osseous system, as in the *coluber scaber* and other serpents, in which true osseous eminences, coated by enamel, pierce the esophagean tunics, and project into the tube; they are attached to about thirty vertebræ, of which they form the inferior spinous process. These are intended to crush the eggs that the serpents feed upon.

"Having established the fact that teeth may spring from bone as well as mucous membrane, Lafosse leads us, where we never suspected, to consider the dental tumors above spoken of as congenital, and he looks on them as having sprung from some rudiment of a maxillary bone. In a word, he looks on the abnormal tooth in question—without offering any plausible explanation—as an aberration in development. He does not class such teeth with the teeth formed in the ovary, &c., but rather with those instances where an extra limb or portion of an extremity is to be met with. It is an accidental excess of parts in an otherwise well-formed body. 'It cannot,' says Lafosse, 'be looked on as an osseous transformation of certain tissues.'

"I have spoken of the case at length, for surgically it is of the very greatest interest. As pathological anatomists, it is our duty to study the laws of disease as well as health. It is praiseworthy to dive into the mysteries of the origin of monsters, but it is essential to adhere to facts and not sacrifice them to theoretical explanations.

"In common with others, I have studied several of these dental tumors. They may spring from several of the bones of the head, but especially from the region of the petrous temporal bone. They may project toward the interior of the cranium, but they more frequently project outwardly. They may be strongly implanted in the bone, or get separated; then they are maintained in their situation by the soft textures around. Their development is not more extraordinary than that of other osseous growths that spring from the cranial or maxillary bones; and their tooth-formed structure (teeth in the region of teeth), is not more wonderful than bony tumors in other parts of the system, whether connected or not with the skeleton."

Prof. William Sewell, President of the British Veterinary Medical Association, at the meeting of that body on May 15, 1838, advanced an interesting theory of the growth of abnormal teeth. It may be true, for after the teeth have attained their full growth, it is reasonable that the dental arteries are less active. But as the teeth continue to grow throughout life, a fact Prof. Sewell does not mention, it is not so reasonable that they even "in a manner *cease*" to act. The professor's remarks are thus reported ("Veterinarian," 1838, "Proceedings Vet. Med. Ass.," p. 199):

"The President begged leave to direct the attention of the meeting to a horse's tooth that had been presented to him. It was a fine specimen of the anomaly occasionally observed in the dental system of the horse —the production of teeth in other places than the alveolar cavities, after the natural teeth had been perfected. The situations which Nature in her wanderings selected were occasionally very singular. He had seen a tooth which grew from the petrous portion of the temporal bone, like a young horn from the forehead of a calf. It formed a hard and seemingly very painful tumor, which was ultimately opened, and the bony substance, which proved to be an almost perfect tooth, extracted. He had seen three or four similar cases in which teeth had been thus produced. When the dental arteries in a manner cease to act—the teeth having attained their full growth—there was a singular predisposition in the neighboring arteries to take on the same action, and teeth, more or less perfect, were formed in parts altogether unconnected with dentition. In this case there were two, one on either side of the forehead."

Surgeon F. Denenbourg makes a detailed report in "The Veterinarian" for 1869 (p. 533) of six cases of dental cyst, five of which he operated on successfully. The first case he treated was in 1837. He confesses that he believed them to be mucous tumors till 1851, when he found a molar tooth perfectly formed. This tooth, which was deposited in an anatomical museum, was as large as a pigeon's egg, and had three roots.

Surgeon C. C. Grice. of New York, makes the following report ("Veterinarian," 1867, p. 392):

"Whether the case the facts of which I am about to communicate will prove of sufficient interest to be presented to the notice of the veterinary profession, or will add anything to the advancement of veterinary pathology. I know not; yet I would be glad to see it inserted in our respectable old journal, 'The Veterinarian,' for I hold it to be the duty of every member of the profession to advance its interests to the best of his ability. I send it because to me it is a very rare case. I have now been in practice more than forty years, and I have not met with anything of the kind before.

"At the request of Mr. Barnum, a merchant of our city and the owner of a breeding-farm in Westchester County, I attended a two-year-old colt, considered to be very valuable, as he comes from trotting stock. Mr. Barnum merely said the colt had a discharge from the base of the near ear, and that it had existed for ten months.

"I found the animal so very shy on account of the previous torturing of his attendants, that I could not approach him; therefore I had to cast him. The introduction of the probe failed to satisfy me that any foreign body existed there; but on dilating the orifice and introducing the most reliable of all probes, my forefinger, I discovered a hard substance, which was firmly attached to the temporal bone and surrounding parts. I could not grasp the substance with the forceps, therefore I used the handle of the instrument as a lever, and after using great force dislodged it. Mr. Barnum picked up something in the grass four or five yards from me, and it proved to be a molar tooth. On examining the wound afterward I found some loose fragments of bone, and on removing them they appeared to be the socket of the tooth.

"I would have sent you a report of this case earlier, but I was desirous of seeing its termination. Mr. Barnum says the parts have entirely healed and left no blemish."

Prof. William Williams advances an interesting theory regarding the cause of dental cysts and also the manner of their formation. He says ("Principles and Practice of Veterinary Surgery," p. 412):

"Cysts containing teeth have been found in the testicles and other parts of the body, but those which are of importance to practical men are found within the antrum. I have seen several cases of this kind, and have extracted teeth from cysts even so high as the base of the ear.

"During life these tumors are distinguishable by more or less disfigurement of the face, by a bulging out of the superior maxillary bone, accompanied in some cases by amaurosis of one eye, succeeded by atrophy of the eye from the pressure of the growing tumor. In other cases these complications are not present, but now and then an abscess forms in the post-orbital region, which will be found on examination to contain a hard body—an imperfect tooth.

"To understand the process by which these tumors are formed, it is necessary to remember that the teeth of all animals belong to and arise from the membranous portion of the digestive canal, and that at a very early period of fetal life a provision is made for the development of the permanent teeth as well as the temporary. This provision, according to Goodsir, is as follows: 'As early as the sixth week of intra-uterine life (human), a groove appears along the border of the future jaws, called the *primitive dental groove*, which is lined by the membrane of the mouth. At the bottom of this groove projections—papillæ—spring up, corresponding in number with the temporary teeth. While the growth of the papillæ is going on, partitions are formed across the grooves, by which they become separated from each other. These partitions subsequently form the bony sockets, thus placing each papilla in a separate cavity. Concurrent with this process, small growths take place upon the membrane of the mouth, just as they dip into the papillary cavity or follicle, which finally, by union with other growths, form a lid which covers the papillæ in a closed sac or bag. Before the final closing of the follicle, a slight folding inward of its lining membrane takes place. This inward folding of the membrane of the primitive groove is for the purpose of forming a new cavity—*the cavity of reserve*—which furnishes a delicate mucous membrane for the future formation of the permanent teeth. The cavity in which the permanent tooth is developed is a mere detachment from the lining of the primitive groove, and in it a papilla is formed in the same way as that of a temporary tooth.'*

"Now, I look on the formation of these tumors as being due to some irregularity in this folding of the lining membrane, by which the 'cavity of reserve' is made up of several folds; that these folds eventually become separated, forming separate cavities of reserve, and that a papilla similar to those of the natural teeth is developed in each cavity. These irregular papillæ are converted into irregular teeth, which, for want of space in the mouth, are forced into the antrum, and may completely block it up, as well as the posterior nasal opening.

"I have classified them as cystic tumors, as at first they are inclosed in sacs or cysts. They soon burst through their investing membrane, however, and form a large tumor, composed entirely of teeth, having a

---

* Compare Professor Goodsir's theory with those advanced by Messrs. Owen, Tomes, Chauveau, and others in the first chapter.

great variety of shapes, and running in different directions. The teeth vary in size, some being very small, while others are nearly as large as a permanent grinder. Each tooth has a pulp cavity, and is composed of the same substances as the natural teeth. Should their removal be desirable, it will be necessary to trephine the superior maxillary sinus and detach them with the forceps."

In the chapter entitled "The Pathology of the Teeth" (the VIII.), Surgeons Bouley and Ferguson, in the course of their memoir on horses' teeth, record some important facts about supernumerary teeth. In one animal the rows of grinders are said to appear double. The facts are given in that particular chapter in preference to the present one in order that the memoir may have a connected reading.

M. Roche Lubin gives the following account of a tooth that he extracted from the upper jaw of a young bull ("Le Zooïatre du Midi," February, 1838):

"On the 14th of April, 1837, I was requested by M. Bonhome, who lives near Rhodez, to extract a tooth which was growing in the middle of the palate of his young bull. The novelty of the thing made me hasten to comply with his request. The animal being secured, I removed the tooth in the usual way. A very considerable hemorrhage followed its extraction, which was performed with some difficulty on account of the tooth being firmly implanted in the palatine arch. It was situated at the middle of the median line, and was of precisely the same character as that of the usual incisor tooth of the ox. This is, I believe, the only case on record, the incisor teeth being wanting in the upper jaw of cattle."

Human beings, like the lower animals, are now and then afflicted with a superfluity of tooth-substance, or at least they have supernumerary teeth. John Hunter says ("The Human Teeth," p. 53):

"We often meet with supernumerary teeth, and this, as well as some other variations, happens oftener in the upper than in the lower jaw, and, I believe, always in the incisors and cuspidati. I have only met with one case of this kind, and it was in the upper jaw of a child about nine months old. The bodies of two teeth, in shape like the cuspidati, were placed directly behind the bodies of the two first permanent incisors; so that there were three teeth in a row, placed behind one another, namely, the temporary incisor, the body of the permanent incisor, and that supernumerary tooth. The most remarkable circumstance was that these teeth were inverted, their points being turned upward and bent, caused by the bone which was above them not giving way to their growth, as the alveolar process does."

The following account of cases of third dentition in human beings is from "Bond's Dental Medicine" (p. 216):

"*Third Dentition.*—A number of well authenticated cases of partial and even complete dentition, occurring in very old persons, are recorded in the books. In one instance, given in the 'Edinburgh Medical Com.' (vol. iii.), the patient, who was sixty years old and entirely toothless, suffered very severely. At the end of twenty-one days from the beginning of his sufferings, however, he was compensated by the appearance of a complete set of new teeth.

"With regard to the constitutional effects of this abnormal dentition, Prof. Harris, who relates two cases as having occurred under his own observation, says: 'It seems that the efforts made by nature for the production of a third complete set of teeth are usually so great that they exhaust the remaining energies of the system, for occurrences of this kind are generally soon followed by death.'"

RETENTION OF DECIDUOUS TEETH.—Miss A. B., aged twenty years, has never shed her deciduous second molars. They are sound and healthy, except one. The first bicuspids have been erupted; the second have not. Would it be proper to extract the temporary teeth?—M. A.

In answer to M. A., in the November, 1881, number of the *Dental Cosmos*, I would reply that from my experience it would be poor practice to extract healthy deciduous molars at that age, merely because they were deciduous, and when *nothing else* indicated such treatment. I have met with many such cases. Sometimes only one or two of the molars are retained; at other times three or four. I know of two sisters, over forty years of age, who have each their four deciduous second molars, and every one perfectly healthy.—*Stormont*.

# CHAPTER VII.

### HORSES' TEETH UNDER THE MICROSCOPE.

#### The Dentinal Tubes, Enamel Fibers, and Cemental Canals Described and Contrasted.

Prof. Richard Owen's description of the microscopical appearance of horses' teeth, like the extracts already made from his works, is both interesting and profound. The teeth described are illustrated in the second volume of the "Odontography," the section of the molar being magnified three hundred linear diameters; that of the incisor, however, is not magnified. In the first volume (pp. 576-7-8) Prof. Owen says:

"The body of the long molar teeth of the horse consists of columns of fine-tubed, unvascular dentine, coated by enamel, which descends in deep folds into the substance of the teeth. The enamel is covered by cement, thickest in the interspaces of the inflected enamel-folds and upon the crowns of the molars, where it is permeated by vascular canals, thinnest on the crowns of the canines and incisors. At the roots of these teeth, and on those developed from the worn-down molars, the dentine is immediately invested by cement.

"In a vertical section of the incisor, as in Plate 136, Fig. 11, the pulp-cavity, contracting as it approaches the vertical enamel-fold, divides near the end of that fold, and extends a little way between it and the periphery of the incisor, or leaves a few medullary canals and a modified thin tract of irregularly formed dentine between the reflected and the outer coat of enamel, but rather nearer the former. Above this tract, near the summit of the crown, the dentinal tubes proceed in a nearly vertical direction, with a gentle sigmoid primary flexure, where they diverge from the perpendicular. Lower down they diverge in opposite directions, curving from the remains of the pulp-fissure toward the outer and the inner enamel, and are described by Retzius as being in the form of the Greek $\varepsilon$; but the course of two distinct series of dentinal tubes, and not of a single tube, is illustrated by this comparison. When the pulp-cavity comes single and central, as at the lower half of the tooth, the tubes diverge to the periphery, with one principal primary curve, convex toward the crown. Each tube is bent in minute secondary gyrations to within a short distance of its peripheral termination, where it is much diminished in size, and is dichotomously branched. The tubes at their beginning form the upper calcified tracts of the pulp-cavity, which usually retain some remnants of that vascular receptacle in the form of medullary canals, and are strongly and irregularly flexuous before they fall into the ordinary primary curves. These tubes, proceeding toward the inner reflected folds of enamel, are more vertical than the tubes going to the periphery.

"A transverse section of the incisor of a young horse or ass, taken across the part marked $a$ in Fig. 11, shows a long oval island of vascular cement in the center, bounded by a border of enamel, with an irregular crenate edge next the cement, and an even edge next the dentine, which is here clearly seen to be divided into an inner and an outer tract by an irregular series of the vascular canals continued from the summit of the pulp-cavity, and by the irregularly tortuous dentinal tubes, which, with the canals, indicate the last converted remnant of the pulp in this part of the crown. The inner tract of dentine next the island of enamel is well defined, and a little broader than the secretion of the enamel itself, and shows the extremities of the tubes cut transversely, which, as before observed, were at this point directed chiefly in the axis of the incisor toward the working surface of the crown. The tubes in the outer tract of dentine, inclining more toward the sides of the tooth, are more obliquely divided, and at the ends of the section they are seen lengthwise, elegantly diverging toward the sides of the section. This tract of dentine is bounded externally by a layer of enamel, one-sixth part thicker than that forming the central island; and the enamel is coated by an outer layer of cement, of its own thickness at the sides, but thinning off at the two ends of the section. The dentinal tubes proceeding from the residuary pulp-tract make strong and irregular curvatures, diverging to include the divided areas of the vascular canals, and in the outer layer, at one side of the section, they describe strong zigzag curves at the middle of the outer division of the dentine.

"The diameter of the dentinal tubes at their central and larger ends is pretty regular, about $\frac{1}{6000}$th of an inch; at the middle of their course, $\frac{1}{8000}$th of an inch, thence decreasing, and very rapidly, after the terminal bifurcations begin. The tubes are separated from one another by intervals varying between once and twice their thickness. In some parts of the dentine of the incisor they are more closely crowded together, especially near their origin from the pulp-cavity. Their secondary gyrations describe a curve of about $\frac{1}{1500}$th of an inch in length. These subside in the slender terminations of the tubes, which bifurcate dichotomously once or twice, and send off small lateral branches near the enamel. The small lateral branches are chiefly visible in the peripheral third part of the tubes, and are sent off at very acute angles, except in the strongly and irregularly bent origins from the pulp-tract. I have never seen these small branches of the dentinal tubes terminating in radiated cells, like those of cement and bone, as Retzius describes; but the peripheral smallest branches near the enamel occasionally dilate into corpuscles much more minute than the radiated cells, as they do in the teeth of most quadrupeds.

"The dentine, as seen in a longitudinal section of the crown of a molar, by a magnifying power of three hundred linear dimensions, is figured at *a*, Plate 137. The tubes are here separated by rather wider interspaces than those of the incisor, and do not decrease in size so rapidly. The convexity of the terminal bend of the tubes is turned toward the summit of the crown. In the incisor, the clear dentinal cells are very small near the peripheral part of the dentine, but increase in size as they approach the pulp-cavity. They are of a sub-circular figure, with bright, transparent lines.

"The central cement in the crown of the incisor is permeated by vascular canals, separated by intervals of from two to three times their own diameter, directed in the middle of the substance in the axis of the tooth, but diverging like rays obliquely toward its periphery.

The clear substance forming the walls of the canals is arranged in concentric layers, the thickness of the walls being about equal or rather less than the area of the canal. The radiated cells, generally of a full oval, sometimes of an angular form, are chiefly dispersed in the interspaces of the vascular canals, and with their long axis parallel with the plane of the layers of the coats. The finer system of tubes radiating from the cells, and corresponding by minute branches from the vascular canals, freely intercommunicate. In the peripheral cement of the incisors examined by me, I found no vascular canals, but only the radiated cells, and the fine tubuli which I have called 'cemental,' and which traverse the cement at right angles to its plane, and communicate with the tubes radiating from the cells. These are more usually elliptical than in the thicker central cement, their long axis being parallel with the borders of the cement. They are most abundant next the enamel, and rarely encroach upon the clear peripheral border of the cement. The exterior coronal cement of the molars (Plate 137, $c$), is as richly permeated by vascular canals ($v$ $v$), as is the central cement of the incisor.

"The enamel-fibers of the horse's incisor are very slender, not exceeding twice the diameter of the dentinal tubes. They extend, with a single sigmoid curve, through the entire thickness of the layer. contiguous fibers curving in opposite directions. The peripheral border, or that next the cement, is everywhere indented with hemispherical pits from $\frac{1}{500}$th to $\frac{1}{2000}$th of an inch in diameter, from four to six of the radiated cells of the cement being often clustered together in the larger depressions. The inner or dentinal border is nearly even and straight; here are seen the short cracks or fissures extending into the enamel. The fibers are rather more wavy in the thicker enamel of the molar teeth (Plate 137, *b*).

"If the enamel is viewed in sufficiently thin sections it is free from those wavy, dusky markings which are produced by the more tortuous fibers of the human enamel; and I have been unable to distinguish any transverse striæ in the fine fibers of that tissue in the horse. The appearance of such is given by thicker sections of the enamel-fibers taken obliquely across them, and is produced by the cut ends of the fibers."

# CHAPTER VIII.

### THE PATHOLOGY OF THE TEETH.

*Importance of the Subject.—Caries caused by Inflamed Pulps, Blows, Virus, and Morbid Diathesis —Supernumerary Teeth and other Derangements.—Trephining the Sinuses.—Gutta Percha as a Filling.—Cleaning the Teeth.—A Diseased Fossil Tooth.*

THE importance of the study of the pathology of the teeth is self-evident, for they not only bear important relations to the general system, but, like all other parts of it, are subject to disease and derangement. The fact that disease of the teeth is involved in more or less mystery, is an argument in favor of the study of the subject, for, to use Surgeon Gamgee's words, it is a "duty to study the laws of disease as well as health," and "it is praiseworthy to dive into the mysteries of the origin of" diseases as well as monsters. It is probably not too much to say that, to the successful surgeon, knowledge of the diseases and derangements of the teeth is indispensable.

In order to facilitate the study of and cast light on the subject, I have brought into juxtaposition, as it were, a summary of the views of a few able men in regard to the cause of caries, &c., which, better still, is followed by the reports of well-known surgeons, who give the results of their experiences in detail.

Dr. G. A. Mills says that when the tone of a tooth can be brought to the point of resistance of the inflammatory process, dentists will have gone a long way in providing against the effects of caries. The dentine decays faster than the enamel.

Prof. Owen says a tooth has no inherent power of reparation; that in growing teeth, with roots not fully formed, the cement is so thin that the Purkinjean cells are not visible. It looks like a fine membrane, and has been described as the periosteum\* of the roots. It increases in thickness with the age of the tooth, and is the seat and origin of what are called *exostoses* of the roots. These growths are subject to the formation of abscesses and all morbid actions of true bone. Of a diseased fossil horse's tooth he says:

"But the cavity had evidently been the result of some inflammatory and ulcerative process in the original formative pulp."

Dr. Boon Hayes says:

"I think it would not be difficult to prove that caries of the teeth more frequently proceeds from inflammation beginning in the pulpal cavity than from any other cause."

Dr. Robley Dunglison says:

"The most common causes of caries are blows, the action of some virus, and morbid diathesis."

---

\* Surgeon John Hughes says: "The periosteum of the teeth is not supplied with blood in the way the same membrane in other parts of the body usually is. It is supplied by means of vessels coming from the pulp of the tooth." If this is true, then it would be easy for inflammation to be conveyed from one to the other.

"Odontonecrosis" is defined by him as "dental gangrene," and "Odontrypy" as "the operation of perforating a tooth to evacuate the purulent matter confined in the cavity of the pulp" (pulpal cavity).

Prof. William Percivall, referring to two diseased grinder teeth (horses'), says:

"They seemed to have been cases which had originated in internal injury."

Surgeons Bouley and Ferguson say:

"In explaining caries of the teeth, we cannot invoke the aid of inflammation and the modifications which it induces in the tissues it attacks; nor can we say that inflammation implies an active circulatory movement, an afflux of liquid, an alteration, nervous derangement, &c."

Possibly the gentlemen were not aware of the inflammation that Prof. Owen says may exist "in the original formative pulp," and of that of "the pulpal cavity"—the pulp in the cavity of a full-grown tooth—mentioned by Drs. Hayes and Dunglison. Are not such inflammations liable to be produced by colds or violent shocks?

Prof. George Varnell, who believes caries of the roots of horses' teeth is usually caused by external violence, says:

"Inflammation of the alveolo-dental periosteum would tend to this result (caries of the roots). When the nutrition of any part of a tooth becomes arrested, decay is likely to follow. When caries begins from within, it is due to arrestation of nutrition, arising perhaps from disease of only a part of the central pulp of the tooth; if from without, it will arise from the periodontal membrane where it meets the gum."

Dr. John Tomes thus describes the conservative action of nature (barricading disease, as it were) when a tooth is affected with caries ("Dental Physiology and Surgery"):

"When a portion of dentine has become dead, it is circumscribed by the consolidation of the adjacent living tissue. The tubes, becoming filled up, are rendered solid, and the circulation is cut off from the dead mass. This consolidation does not go on gradually from without inward, keeping in advance of the decay, but occurs at intervals. It seems that successive portions of dentine lose their vitality, and that the contiguous living portions become consolidated."

Prof. M. H. Bouley and Surgeon P. B. Ferguson are the joint authors of a memoir on horses' teeth, which fills thirty or more pages of "The Veterinarian" for 1844. The substance of the part which relates to the pathology and dentistry of the teeth is as follows:*

"1. *Anomalies in the Number of the Teeth.*—Sometimes, but very rarely, we meet with supernumerary grinders in the horse. The anomaly may be caused by the persistence of the temporary teeth, the development of abnormal teeth on one or both sides of the arcades (rows of teeth), and the cutting of a greater

---

* The phraseology of Messrs. Bouley and Ferguson's memoir has been more or less changed and the matter somewhat condensed and rearranged. The surgeons' golden ideas deserve to be set forth in clearer and more forcible language than they receive at their own hands, and it is believed that some improvement has been made.

number of permanent teeth than should naturally exist. In the latter case it is necessary to admit the existence of a greater number of dental bulbs than is normal. We saw some time ago, at the consultation of the Veterinary College in Alfort,* a horse which, to use the words of its owner, 'had a double row of teeth in the upper jaw.'

"Sometimes the supernumerary tooth is situated in one or the other jaw, in front of the normal range of grinders, without having a corresponding tooth in the opposite jaw; at other times it is situated either within or without the arcade. The latter anomaly is caused more frequently by the deviation of a normal than by the addition of a supernumerary tooth. In the first instance it is not long before mastication is interfered with. The tooth, by its growth, which is not counteracted by wear, finally reaches the opposite jaw, lacerating the mucous membrane and contusing and sometimes fracturing the bone itself. In the second instance, the tooth, if within the arcade, is an obstacle to the tongue; if without, to the cheek. Besides these evil effects, supernumerary teeth cause irregularity in the arcades, and consequently prevent the exact apposition of the normal teeth. They interfere also with the action of the lower jaw. Hence irregularity in the friction and wear of the teeth follows, the result being that the performance of the all-important function of mastication is almost stopped.

"2. *Anomalies in the Form of the Arcades.*—The upper rows of grinder teeth form two curves, opposed by their concavities, while the lower rows form two

---

* A city of France—Prof. Bouley's home. Surgeon Ferguson, an Englishman, was attached to the Paris British Legation.

nearly straight lines, which converge as they descend toward the symphysis of the chin. These (the curves and lines) may be, owing, in some cases, to congenital conformation, very irregular. Sometimes, in fact, the curves of the upper jaw are effaced; at other times, and most frequently, the lines of the lower jaw are incurvated within the upper arcades. The deformities may exist singly or together. The result is that, in the approach of the jaws, the relation is not identically established between the surfaces of friction, and the result of this, in turn, is an irregularity of wear and an abnormal development of the borders of the tables (the crowns of the teeth), within in the lower jaw, without in the upper.

"3. *Exuberance of particular parts of the Dental Apparatus.*—(A.) The upper grinders are wider than the lower, so that in order to cause friction in their entire thickness, a lateral movement of the lower jaw is required. Sometimes, perhaps because the movement is not effected throughout the entire limits of the segment of the circle, the outer borders of the upper teeth do not wear sufficiently, and therefore become elevated and sharp. At other times it is the inner borders of the lower teeth that project. In the former case the cheeks suffer; in the latter, the tongue.

"In rare cases the tables, which present a normal inclination *inverse* in the two jaws, at length form planes very oblique. The obliquity is sometimes so great that the internal borders of the lower teeth are very elevated, while the external is almost level with the gums. The inverse effect manifests itself at the upper jaw. The consequence is that the half-masticated food slips into the pouch of the cheek.

"There is in the museum of the College at Alfort a horse's head in which this deformity may be seen in its greatest degree. The tables of the teeth at the right side form planes so much inclined that they close together like the blades of shears. As there was no friction to wear the teeth down, they grew to the hight of three inches. The fourth and fifth teeth of the right side of this rare anatomical specimen are absent. Perhaps they were carious. The rarefied and spongy tissue of the socket-bones indicate the seat of an alteration—probably caries—which was the point of departure of the general tumefaction. The last tooth, by its oblique direction toward the empty sockets, indicates that the loss of the teeth occurred during the life of the animal, some time perhaps prior to its death. The defect of the right side doubtless forced the animal to use the left for the purposes of mastication. In such cases the teeth that do not wear grow till they reach their respective opposite jaws, even when those at the opposite side of the mouth are in exact contact, an anomaly never produced in the normal state. The function of mastication operates according to the obliquity of contact, and a parallelism is established by friction between the tables which normally would be superposed.

"This appears to us to be the only interpretation of the facts, and we have observed two analogous examples in living horses, but we did not think to ascertain whether the deformity of an entire arcade was owing to defect of a grinder or to disease of the bone. The solution of the question would be an important acquisition to the science of dental pathology.

"(B.) There is another kind of deformity of the arcades not very uncommon. The lower teeth wear out more rapidly than the upper, the cause of which is perhaps owing to the superiority of the latter in size and strength. The crown surface of the lower rows is slightly concave, the upper rows slightly convex. The result is that the lower center teeth are sometimes worn to their sockets, which renders the mastication of hard food impossible. At first, however, there is no interference with mastication, and it is usually only in old age that the deformity reaches its worst stage. There is no remedy for the defect, *but its progress may be retarded by the use of soft food.*\*

"(C.) Lack of regularity in the length of the rows becomes the cause, in horses a little advanced in age, of a peculiar deformity in the first upper and the last lower grinders. Generally the upper range passes that of the lower by some lines, the first upper grinder lapping over; but sometimes the case is the reverse, the last lower grinder projecting beyond the last upper. The projecting part of the tooth grows till it reaches the opposite jaw, when, unless it is filed or chiseled off, the most serious consequences will follow.

"(D.) When a tooth is entirely deficient, the opposite tooth grows till it fills the void; then, no remedy being applied, the work of destruction begins. If a tooth is only partly deficient, no matter whether it be from fracture, caries, or arrestation of growth, it is gradually destroyed by the opposite tooth. When it is the first upper grinder that is deficient, the first lower acts on the palatine vault like a battering-ram. 'I have seen,' says Solleysel (1669), 'a mule that had a lower grinder of extreme length, the upper tooth being absent. The palate was pierced to the thickness of a

---

\* The italicized words are mine.—*C.*

finger, which caused the animal great difficulty when he drank.'

"*4. Caries of the Teeth.*—The grinder teeth of horses are more frequently affected with a profound alteration of their substance than is generally believed. The disease is called *Caries;* it may not, however, be strictly analogous to caries of the bones, for the bones are vascular, while the teeth have neither vessels nor nerves. Caries of the bones implies an active labor, in which the vascular apparatus plays an important part. It is a phenomenon of interstitial suppuration, under the influence of the inflammation which has set the capillary system of the organ in play. In explaining caries of the teeth, however, we cannot invoke the aid of inflammation and the modifications it induces in the tissues it attacks; nor can we say that inflammation implies an active circulatory movement, an afflux of liquid, an alteration, nervous derangement, &c. If the teeth are living, the laws which govern their vitality are entirely unknown to us.\* How, then, penetrate into the secrets of the alterations which they undergo, when the conditions of their normal existence are enveloped in obscurity? Neither is it possible to resolve the question as to the essence of the affection designated by the name of caries. Therefore we design to make known only the different modes of expression relative to it.

"Caries usually attacks the dentine of the crown of the teeth, between two folds of enamel. The dentine becomes of a brownish or blackish color, and dissemi-

---

\* It should be borne in mind that the above views were enunciated more than a third of a century ago. The gentlemen probably say too much. Compare with Dr. Hayes's views as recorded on page xxii.

nates an offensive odor *sui generis*, which perhaps is as much owing to the putrefaction of the saliva in the cavity as to the decomposition of the dentine. The decay progresses between the folds of enamel, and the latter substance, notwithstanding its great density, takes on the blackish tint of the dentine and becomes sufficiently softened to allow of its being cut by a sharp instrument. Sometimes even the planes of the enamel dissolve, and then the cubic mass of the tooth becomes so much decayed that it resembles a deep cavity, the parietes of which are formed by the planes of enamel laid bare by the caries. Sometimes caries attacks the tooth on one of its four side surfaces; at other times the root is attacked; but wherever its primitive seat may be, the blackish veins always extend into the dentine, and thus isolate the plies of enamel.

"Carious teeth rarely preserve either their form or volume. They become hypertrophied at their roots, but the effect does not manifest itself until the disease —having undermined all the layers of dentine in its course—has penetrated the root. When the caries has penetrated to the socket, the alveolo-dental membrane becomes irritated by the contact of decayed matter, increases its secretion, and deposits a thick layer of osseous matter in the circumference of the root of the tooth, which concretes irregularly upon the normal layers. The deposition does not, however, always take place in the circumference of the root, for in some cases it is only at isolated places that the secretion of the alveolo-dental membrane occurs. Then the root presents a succession of large osseous tubercles, which bar the tooth in, rendering its extraction very difficult. When the irritation has been from the first sufficiently active to cause suppurative inflammation, the **normal** secretion is suspended, and pus collects in the alveolar cavity, around the root, which then ceases to augment in volume. In the former case, however, the root, augmented in volume, can no longer be contained in the cavity, the walls of which are expanded by its wedge-like action, which accounts for the extreme pain in the adjacent parts, and the particular alterations in the osseous tissues. The osseous tissue tumefies, and suppuration is established in the interior of the socket; the membrane is partly destroyed, which leaves the bone bare and exposed to the maceration of pus and the irritating contact of the morbid matter that continually penetrates into the socket by the dental fistula; the bony tissue sphacelates upon the borders, where its substance is the most compact, and its spongy tissue, which forms the bottom of the cavity, soon becomes the seat of an interstitial suppuration— that is to say, in fact, of veritable caries. The swelling may now extend throughout the entire extent of the maxillary bone, and thus render mastication impossible.

"It may now be seen, an alteration of this nature being set in action, how the phenomena of the nutrition of bone may be modified in their direction to the point of producing *osteo-sarcoma*.

"Caries of the roots of any of the lower grinders may be complicated with lesions of the jaw, for the lower jaw is continuous in its entire extent. In the upper jaw the phenomena are in principle the same, but the contiguous nasal cavities and sinuses induce complications the study of which is important. It is also important to take into consideration the position of the diseased tooth, in order to appreciate the extent of the lesions which a simple caries may produce.

"The two first upper grinder teeth are separated from the nasal cavities by a thin bone, which is easily eaten through. When caries attacks their roots, the inflammation extends itself to the membrane lining these cavities, and a perforation of the osseous partition may establish communication between the mouth and the nose. Under the influence of interstitial suppuration, the osseous membrane is destroyed to an enormous extent. The aliments pass through the dental fistula into the nose and are expelled by it along with the product of the morbid secretion of the pituitary membrane.

"The third grinder is situated near the maxillary sinuses, from which the root is separated by a thin diaphragm. It deserves to be specially noticed on account of an anatomical peculiarity, which renders caries of this tooth very much to be dreaded. We refer to the position of large fasciæ (bundles) of the superior maxillary branch of the fifth pair of nerves, which make their exit upon the face by the submaxillary foramen, and which are placed immediately over the root of this tooth. It is easy to imagine the pain that may follow nervous complications in caries of the roots of the third grinder.

"The position of the fourth, fifth, and sixth grinder teeth, immediately below the vast maxillary sinuses, from which their roots are separated by thin osseous partitions. gives to caries of these teeth, and to the complications which it induces, a special character, which demands that we should speak of it somewhat in detail. These teeth communicate with the sinuses as easily as the first and second do with the nose; but the case is far worse for the horse, there being so little outlet for the pus.

"When the disease has penetrated the roots, and has induced the usual inflammation, the thin partitions that separate them from the sinuses do not resist very long. Destroyed by the dilatory effort of the hypertrophied root and the influence of the caries, the altered matters of the mouth have free access into the sinuses. Under the influence of their contact, the membrane of the sinuses irritates, vascularizes, and thickens by a serous infiltration in the early stage. Then, the primitive cause of this modification continuing, the membrane hypertrophies somewhat, and in a short time, owing to its vascular system being richly developed by inflammation, large vegetations of the nature of polypi are elevated upon it. These, on account of the incessant augmentation of their volume, fill the sinuses and cause a swelling of their walls.

"When the membrane of the sinuses has become the seat of an abnormal vegetation, an abundant quantity of purulent matter is secreted, the more liquid part of which drains out through the conduits leading to the nasal cavities, while the more concrete part remains in the sinuses. It then, according as it loses its serosity, undergoes a transformation, and finally displays the aspect of cadaveric grease, which it also resembles in its repugnant odor. There is a great analogy between the disease that causes this particular lesion and that of glanders.

"*Symptomatology.*—The first symptom that indicates a derangement of the dental apparatus is a difficulty in mastication. The animal, excited by hunger, seizes the food with avidity. The motions of the lower jaw, however, are made with a sort of hesitation, and often only at one side. The imperfectly masticated hay, which on that account will not pass through the narrow pharynx, is dropped into the manger in the form of cuds or flattened pellets. The nose is plunged into the feed, over which the animal fumbles and nibbles, but of which it eats little.

"The insufficiency of nutrition soon produces a baneful effect on the whole economy. The coat tarnishes, becoming dry and staring; the least exertion makes the animal sweat; it is heedless of the whip; the mucous membranes become discolored; the pulse weakens, and cold infiltrations sometimes appear in the extremities. To see an animal thus suddenly transformed, one is apt to mistake the true cause and attribute it to the influence of some grave organic disturbance.

"These symptoms are common to the different diseases and derangements of the dental apparatus, and are sufficient to lead to a positive diagnosis. The diagnosis, however, can only be precisely determined when the mouth shall have been examined, for by this means we perceive the particular signs of each of the alterations that opposes the function of mastication. The mouth may be kept open by a *speculum oris*, or even by drawing out the free portion of the tongue, which should be held by the thumb and the third and fourth fingers, the index being placed between the inner side of the upper lip and the gum, at the space between the grinders and the tushes, while the other hand is left free to aid the inspection by taxis.

"If the derangement be the result of an exuberance of a tooth, vicious inclination or projections of the tables, fractured teeth, swollen sockets, &c., the sight is ordinarily sufficient to detect it, for the teeth are, besides, frequently soiled by the greenish remains of food at the affected part, and often even the cheek is filled with an accumulation of malground food. The mouth should be cleaned with water, in order that the defect may be more plainly seen; if, however, on account of its being situated far back in the mouth and the motions of the base of the tongue from side to side intercepting the view, its nature cannot be discovered with the eye, it will be necessary to resort to the sense of touch. The mouth being held open by the speculum oris, or some other firmly-fixed apparatus, the fingers should be passed rapidly within and without the arcades, but never on them, because of the danger of having them crushed: whatever may be the degree of forced dilatation of the mouth, there can never be much separation of the jaws in the region of the last grinders; besides the animal can lessen it by pressure.

"When the buccal membrane has been excoriated by the contact of irregularly-worn teeth, the gums inflamed, the jawbones contused, and the latter sphacelate or suppurate, there are some modifications of the general symptoms. The animal loses its appetite, becomes dull, 'crest-fallen,' and agitated with febrile disturbance, however little the heart of the inflammation may be extended. The saliva, which dribbles from the mouth, is stringy, and, when mixed with pus, fetid; the mouth is hot and its membrane injected; there is a turgescence of the gum at the point of inflammation; a tumefaction of the bone, with a grayish tint at the point where it is denuded and about to exfoliate, or else fistulæ abut into the heart of the suppuration in the spongy tissue of the jaw.

"*Particular Symptoms of Caries.*—Caries of the grinder teeth is characterized by peculiar symptoms, some of which are common to the teeth in general, while others belong to some grinders in particular.

To give precision to the diagnosis, the position of the teeth should be taken into consideration. Besides the symptoms common to all disorders of the teeth, caries in general presents as diagnostic signs—

"1. A fetor very remarkable and *sui generis* of the mouth, and of the saliva which humefies it.

"2. Dribbling of an abundant and stringy saliva from the mouth.

"3. Existence on one of the faces of the tooth, and principally upon its crown, either of a blackish spot or a large cavity of the same color, according to the extent of the disease.

"4. The extreme pain that the animal evinces when the tooth is struck.

"If the disease is of long standing, and especially if it has arisen from the side of the root, in addition to the foregoing modifications and complications, other and more special symptoms manifest themselves. The bone tumefies and the animal evinces pain when it is pressed by the fingers; the gums are affected with turgescence, and bleed from the least contact; all the buccal mucous membrane reflects a red tint, and in the meantime fever sets in, manifesting itself by all its ordinary and general symptoms.

"Caries of the first and second upper grinders may, as already explained, be complicated with lesions of the nasal cavities. Then the pituitary membrane irritates and secretes abundant mucosities, but at one side only, with which the food becomes mixed, giving it a green tint, but very different from the secretions of glanders. The case is different, however, in the complications induced by caries of the last grinders. In fact there is such a close resemblance between the symptomatic expressions of the nose following caries of these teeth and chronic glanders, that error and confusion are common. It is therefore highly important to distinguish these diseases, so essentially different in their causes and effects.

"When the membrane lining the sinuses has become diseased, followed by the secretion of pus and polypus growths, a jettage is established at one side of the nose. It is white, lumpy, and abundant, and is augmented in quantity by exercise. The lymphatic ganglions become engorged and hard, but remain indolent, and generally roll under the finger. The zygomatic tables of the upper part of the superior maxillary and nasal bones swell at the region of the affected sinuses, and give a dull sound to percussion.*

---

* Prof. Varnell says: "I am not aware that any animal suffers from diseases of the sinuses of the head to the same extent as the horse. The sinuses differ in size in different breeds, and in individual horses of the same breed. I need scarcely point out the necessity of bearing this fact in mind in forming diagnoses of obscure diseases in this region of the head. In certain cases it is not only important to ascertain whether the sinuses contain anything abnormal, but also the nature and extent of the morbific matter. Percussion with the ends of the fingers is one mode of obtaining this information. Both sides of the head should be struck, and the sound produced in one part compared with that in another, and with what it is in health. I would recommend students to become familiar with these various sounds. They will be found to differ, according to the magnitude of the sinuses, in the same way that a large empty cask, when struck, will differ in sound from a small one. It will also be well to educate the ear to the character of the sounds produced by percussing the sinuses in differently formed heads. * * * The sinuses, strictly speaking, are air cavities, which communicate freely with each other, and by means of a

"At the first appearance of this group of symptoms one is apt to suspicion the existence of glanders, but a careful examination will prove it to be unfounded. On examining the nasal cavity, the lining membrane will be seen to be smooth, polished, and uniformly rosy, with its normal follicular openings, and on unfolding the superior wing of the nostril, the salient border of the cartilage presents a neat and polished surface, *without any little pimples or morbid tint*. Now, we know that in glanders, even of the sinuses, which is often unaccompanied by cankers or other ulcerations, it is in those places certain specific morbid signs may be recognized, which, although very superficial and with difficulty seen by the eye, are nevertheless of great value in the diagnosis. Such, for instance, are the peculiar aspect of the salient border of the wing of the nostril, with its vivid red tint, the small superficial erosions of the lining membrane, entirely hidden under the fold of the cartilage, and those small granular projections called tubercles. In the jettage from caries nothing of this kind exists. There is a marked difference in the odor too; in caries the odor is exceedingly fetid, while in glanders it is almost null.

"If, after this attentive examination, the surgeon is still in doubt as to the specific nature of the nasal dis-

---

small opening, with the nasal passage also. This opening is situated at the supero-posterior part of the middle meatus, and is guarded by an imperfect valve, which, when pressed upon from within, either partially or wholly closes it. It may also be closed by the mucous membrane being thickened by disease. Internally the sinuses are partially divided into compartments by thin osseous plates, and are lined by a slightly vascular membrane, which is continuous with that of the nasal passage, but is not so thick nor so vascular."

charge, it will disappear and give place to a true diagnosis when he has examined the mouth and has had time to weigh and compare all the facts in connection with the case.

"It is more especially relative to diseases of the teeth that is recognized the truth of the old maxim in surgery, *Sublatâ causâ, tollitur effectus.*" (The cause being removed, the effect ceases.)

For putting irregular teeth in order, the surgeons recommend the use of a coarse, six-inch file, with a handle from twenty to twenty-four inches long. However, they say that in their day it was customary among the "vulgar" to make the horse *chew a rasp!* The process, which they describe, referring among other things to the difficulty of getting the rasp precisely opposite the projections, is too slow, as they admit, to be practicable; besides it is about as difficult to compel a horse to chew as to compel him to drink.

For the removal of supernumerary grinder teeth or the shortening of natural ones that have grown beyond the level of the other teeth, they recommend the use of a chisel and a hammer; two or three well-directed blows with the latter are usually sufficient to cut the largest tooth in two. The surgeon requires an assistant or "striker." In the case of the first grinder, the blows should be light, otherwise the tooth would be loosened in its socket. In the case of the last grinder, "it is necessary for the operator to be perfectly master of the chisel at the moment of its being struck, for, in escaping, it might strike against the velum palati (soft palate) and cut it through."

In performing these operations they prefer that the horse should be in a standing position, as when in a lying position there is danger of his swallowing the fragments of the teeth. If it is necessary, however, to cast the horse, they recommend that the head rest on the occiput, the operators being as expeditious as possible, to prevent the animal from swallowing the fragments. As the nose points up, the surgeon would have to be expeditious indeed in order to prevent the horse from being drenched, as it were, with tooth-fragments.

The surgeons next describe an interesting case of dental surgery, in the performance of which the bone-forceps were used to remove the tushes. They say:

"It sometimes happens that the fleshy and bony structures of the mouth are not well proportioned, and when the animal is put to work evil consequences result, especially if the tongue is too large for the space between the branches of the jaws. A remarkable case of this kind lately came under our observation in a horse owned by the Earl of Clonmel. The animal, a remarkably fine one, was a very hard 'puller,' in consequence of the bit not coming in sufficient contact with the sensitive bars. The space between the tushes was too narrow for the tongue, which, after the animal had been ridden with restraint by a horse-breaker, was cut nearly through at each side. The consequence was the tongue became swollen to an enormous extent, and as the tushes increased the irritation, their removal became necessary. They were cut off to a level with the gums with the bone-forceps, the tongue was scarified and bathed with a cold lotion, and the animal was fit for work at the end of a week.

"Perhaps at first it may seem better practice in such cases to extract the tushes entirely. But when the length and obliquity of their roots and the fact of their being situated in the weakest part of the jaw are considered, it is plain that such a procedure would in all probability be followed by the most serious results, such as fracture of the jaw, osteo-sarcoma, &c., the former having happened under our own observation."

The surgeons recommend (as any intelligent person would) the removal of supernumerary or abnormal incisor teeth. When the tooth is without the normal range it interferes with the prehensile function of the lips; when within, it interferes with the tongue. The former, they say, may either be cut off with the bone-forceps or extracted. In the latter case, however, they prefer to cut them off, but admit that some teeth require extraction, for which the use of the crank-forceps is recommended.

The *Treatment of Caries* is the next subject considered. "The only remedy for caries," the surgeons say, "in the great majority of cases, is the extraction of the tooth. If we were called on to treat the disease at its beginning, cauterizing the black spot would check its progress; but when the dental bulb has been attacked, the extraction of the tooth is the only remedy."

The instrument recommended for extracting teeth is the forceps, and under ordinary circumstances, the surgeons say, fracture of the jaws ought not to occur. They mention as useful instruments the key invented by M. Garengeot, the mouth-screw by M. Plasse, and the lever-forceps by Prof. Simonds, but say.

"Instances occur in which the carious tooth cannot be seized by any of these instruments. For example, when the last upper grinder is diseased, it is sometimes impossible to dilate the mouth sufficiently to slide the instrument between it and the corresponding lower tooth. Besides, the tongue, however firmly it may be held outside the mouth, has still the power to displace the instrument by the energy of the undulatory movements at its base. Again, the back grinders, having ordinarily shorter bodies than the others, afford less hold for the instrument. In some cases they afford no hold at all, as their bodies are worn almost to a level with the gums.

"Lastly, in some cases the exostosis of the root of the tooth is so great that it is, as it were, wedged in the socket, and resists all efforts to extract it. What is to be done? The disease may lead to grave local complications and dangerous general disorders. In such a case we would recommend trephining the diseased sinus and punching the tooth into the mouth. This operation being very unusual, and the observance of some rules requisite for practicing it, we will consider it somewhat in detail.

"If, as sometimes happens, the swelling over the sinus is indistinct, it would be well to be guided by a prepared head, in order to apply the trephine in the exact place, which is above the diseased root. A large V or crucial incision should be made, and the trephine manipulated till the sinus is laid open. The opening should be extensive rather than confined; it is more convenient to apply upon the parietes of the sinuses three crowns of the trephine, tangent reciprocally at their circumferences; then, by the aid of a sharp instrument and a small hammer, the angles may be removed.

"As soon as the mucous membrane of the cavity has been laid bare, the change it has undergone may be seen, and also the vegetations springing from it. At the bottom of the sinus, toward the alveolar border of the jaw, among the vegetations, is a hard, granulated, dry surface, resistant to the touch, of a grayish tint, and analogous to sphacelated bone. This is the summit of the root of the tooth.

"The surgeon then arms himself with an iron punch, rounded at the point, which he applies to the root in the sinus, and having further separated the jaws by a few turns of the speculum oris, commands an assistant to strike *short*, hard blows, the surgeon looking at the tooth to see the effect of each blow. Usually the tooth soon gives way, and falls into the mouth generally in two fragments, according to the direction of the caries. Sometimes, however, from the length of the tooth, it cannot be punched entirely into the mouth, being stopped by the opposite lower tooth; but it may be wrenched out with a pair of long pincers, the handles of which should be separated to increase the power of the operator. When the operation is terminated, the vegetations of the mucous membrane, as far as they can be reached, must be excised. To stop the hemorrhage, and to modify the state of the membrane, pledgets of tow, moistened with a diluted solution of nitric acid, or some other caustic, should be applied.

"It is really extraordinary with what rapidity the structural breaches resulting from this operation are restored by the reparatory efforts of the organic economy. The first time we performed the operation we doubted the animal's recovery. The sinuses, laid open by a breach nearly two inches and a half in diameter, communicated with the mouth by an enormous opening, the root of the tooth having acquired nearly three times its normal volume. The lining membrane of the maxillary sinuses, and the frontal also, had suffered the transformation already described to its greatest degree. And, finally, it required efforts almost beyond belief to loosen the tooth and force it from its socket. Still the animal made a good recovery.

"The treatment following the operation should be as follows: Assiduous attention to cleanliness is necessary from the first. On the first day the animal should be deprived of all solid or fibrous food; in fact, a little thin gruel is all it requires, and the mouth should be gargled with an acidulated fluid even after its use. The fluid may be applied with an ordinary syringe. Bleeding is often required, the quantity of blood to be abstracted depending on the energy of the reaction following the operation.

"On the day after the operation the dressing should be raised. The interior of the sinus, cauterized with nitric acid, reflects a blackish tint. The odor is repugnant, and there are generally some remains of putrid alimentary matters, mixed with clots of blood, in the sinus. Detergents, such as Labarraque's chlorinated solution of soda, mixed with a gentian wine, should be injected into the sinus and the mouth cleaned with acid gargles; a firm pledget of chlorinated tow should be introduced into the socket, to prevent anything passing from the mouth to the sinus. The regimen should consist of gruel only, the gargles to be used often during the day.

"On the second day the borders of the sinus will be a little swollen. Reparatory work has begun in the cauterized membrane; the eschars detach themselves, exposing a rosy surface of favorable aspect to the view. The odor is less repugnant. Continue the aromatic detergent injections, the same food, with the addition of a little bran, and gargle often. As suppuration begins to establish itself, the dressings should be renewed two or three times during the twenty-four hours.

"It is not our intention to indicate the progress of the wound and the attention it demands from day to day. The tumefied bones and other structures in the region of the wound proportionally lessen, and the membrane of the sinus takes on a uniformly rosy tint and the glistening, humid aspect proper to a mucous membrane. The nasal flux finally ceases, the matter that may be secreted finding an outlet through the alveolus into the mouth. The opening made by the trephine contracts itself by degrees, but in extreme cases, like the one we have described, it is never sufficient to entirely repair the structures cut away. It may be hidden, however, by a leather or metallic plate, attached to the check of the bridle."

The surgeons claim that the resort to this severe mode of extracting teeth is justified by the success of the operation and its concomitant results, namely, the advantage of injecting the sinuses and preventing unhealthy secretions by them, and the stopping of the discharge from the nose, which had aroused suspicion of glanders. They further say—and a better argument in favor of veterinary dentistry could not well be advanced—that they believe glanders is often caused by the neglect of diseased teeth, and "that the *modus operandi* of its production in such cases may be explained on the ground of the absorption of pus by the constitution."

Of trephining the sinuses they further say:

"We have treated many cases of caries successfully by simply trephining the frontal and maxillary sinuses and injecting detergents; but in a far greater number the treatment has been unsuccessful.* Yet we believe that if, in addition to trephining, the teeth had been extracted, and a communication established between the sinus and the mouth, the results would have been more favorable.

"Monsieur Delafond, in his memoir on the evulsion of the teeth, published in 1831, says the operation of trephining is only practicable in the case of the three first grinders, it being necessary in the case of the three last to make an incision through the zygomatico-maxillaris muscle and the nervous plexus which is formed on it. We, on the contrary, claim that the fifth pair of nerves will be injured in operating on the three first teeth, but that there will be little injury to the muscle in the case of the three last."

The memoir concludes as follows:

"*Caries Attacking the Maxillary Bone after the Extraction of the Teeth.*—When caries of a tooth has induced consecutively interstitial suppuration of the spongy tissue of the socket, it is possible that, even after the extraction of the tooth, the disease may attack the bone. Then, more than ever, may we dread the tumefaction of the tissues and sarcomatous alterations, which are ordinarily the result of persistent suppuration in the areolæ of the spongy substance of the bones. To prevent these dangerous consequences, the socket should be cauterized with the actual cautery,

---

* "Sinuses that may have formed by the matter from abscesses in the alveolar processes eating its way through the wall of the alveolus, and which may open either on some part of the face or within the mouth, are seldom treated with the success one could desire."—*Prof. George Varnell.*

and, if it is practicable, a counter opening by trephining should be made. In some cases in our practice this mode of treatment produced the most satisfactory results. If, however, on account of the circumstances of the case, the actual cautery cannot be used, a strong solution of argenti nitras, applied with pledgets of tow or lint, may be substituted.

"*Complications of Operations on the Mouth.*—One of the most ordinary and serious complications of operations on the mouth is the excoriation of the 'bars' by the friction of the speculum oris. The denuded bone often exfoliates, rendering the horse unfit for work for a month or more. The evil may be avoided by enveloping the transverse bars of the speculum with tow or some other elastic material, and by being expeditious in operating. The hemorrhage, which is never abundant enough to be serious, may be checked by pledgets of tow, wet with a solution of either nitric or sulphuric acid.

"*Regimen.*—The regimen in extreme cases of caries has already been indicated in the account of the case of trephining for caries and exostosis of the root of a grinder. In addition to well-boiled gruel, mixed or unmixed with bran, carrots and similar food will be found beneficial." *

---

\* As horses with defective, diseased, or worn-out teeth require soft or ground food, a few extracts from the article on "Food" in Prof. Youatt's work entitled "The Horse" (p. 132) and other sources will not be out of place here: "Oatmeal gruel constitutes one of the most important articles of diet for the sick horse. Few grooms make good gruel. It is either not boiled long enough, or a sufficient quantity is not used. The proportions should be a pound of meal to a gallon of water. It should be constantly stirred till it boils, and for five minutes afterward. Carrots, according to Stewart's 'Stable Economy,' are a good

Prof. George Varnell, of the Royal Veterinary College of London, the author of a series of articles "On substitute for grass, and in sick or idle horses render corn unnecessary. They improve the state of the skin. At first they are slightly diuretic and laxative, but the effect lessens with use. Half a bushel is a large daily allowance. Swedish turnips and raw potatoes are useful foods. Raw potatoes, sliced and mixed with chaff, may be given to advantage, but it is better to boil or steam them, as purging rarely ensues. For horses recovering from sickness, barley in the form of malt is serviceable as tempting the appetite and recruiting the strength. It is best given in mashes, water somewhat below the boiling heat being poured upon it, and the vessel kept covered for half an hour. Rye is used in Germany, but generally cooked as bread, which is made from the whole flour and bran. It is not unusual in traveling through some parts of Germany and Holland to see the postilions help themselves and their horses from the same loaf. In some northern countries peameal is frequently used, not only as food, but as a remedy for diabetes. Linseed, raw, ground, or boiled, is sometimes given to sick horses. Half a pint may be mixed with the feed every night. It is supposed to be useful in cases of catarrh. It is very useful for a cough, but it is too nutritious for a fever. For a cough it should be boiled and given in a bran mash, to which two or three ounces of coarse sugar may be added. Tares, cut after the pods are formed, but some time before the seeds are ripe, lucern, and sainfoin are useful foods. Of the former the variety known as vicia sativa is the best."

On page 511 Prof. Youatt says "some greedy horses habitually swallow their food without properly grinding it." As a remedy he recommends that chaff be mixed with the corn, oats, or beans, which, being too hard and sharp to be swallowed without chewing, compels the horse to masticate his food. He says: "Chaff may be composed of equal quantities of clover or meadow hay and wheaten, oaten, or barley straw, cut in pieces of a quarter or a half an inch in length, and mixed well together. The allowance of corn, oats, or beans is added afterward, and mixed with the chaff. Many farmers very properly bruise the oats and beans. The whole oat is apt to slip out of the chaff and be lost,

Some of the Diseases Affecting the Facial Region of the Horse's Head" ("Veterinarian," 1866–67), and other productions, has made the disorders of horses' teeth a study, and has aided somewhat in clearing the "mystery" that Surgeon Gowing believes will "to a certain extent always remain," for he has succeeded in casting some light on the ætiology of a tooth's greatest enemy—caries. His suggestion as to plugging teeth with gutta-percha is novel, and in some cases might be practicable. However, would not cement, which gives such perfect satisfaction in human dentistry, be preferable? It is not expensive, and can be as readily introduced into a cavity as gutta-percha; besides, as the cavity must first be thoroughly cleaned (no matter which is used), its use in the end might save time and the tooth be much longer preserved. A horse's tooth that can be got at conveniently, ought to be filled as easily and, in decay of its neck, perhaps as successfully as a human tooth. Prof. Varnell's views are in substance as follows ("Veterinarian," 1867):

"Caries of the roots of the grinder teeth is rare and generally very difficult to account for. I think that, in the majority of cases, it depends upon external vio-

For old horses, and for those with defective teeth, chaff is peculiarly useful, and for both classes the grain should be broken as well as the fodder. The proportions are eight pounds of oats and two of beans to twenty of chaff."

Concerning swallowing without grinding Prof. Youatt further says: "In cases of this kind the teeth should be examined. Some of them may be unduly lengthened, particularly the first of the grinders, or their ragged edges may wound the cheek. In the former case the horse cannot properly masticate his food; in the latter he will not, for horses, as too often occurs in sore throat, would rather starve than put themselves to much pain."

lence, although we are not always able to trace it to such a cause. Inflammation of the alveolo-dental periosteum, especially where it surrounds the root or roots of a tooth, would tend to this result. Other causes may produce the same effect. Indeed, whenever or however effected, when the nutrition of any part of a tooth ceases, decay is likely to follow. When caries begins from within, it is due to cessation of nutrition, arising perhaps from disease of only a part of the central pulp of the tooth. If from without, it arises from the periodontal membrane where it meets the gum.

"Caries of the cervix (neck) of the tooth is much more common than it is in the root; still it does not occur in more than one horse in five hundred. The question will naturally be asked, To what does this tendency to decay belong? Under such circumstances are we not forced to the conclusion that it must depend either upon a defective structure of the tooth, or that the dentine, enamel, and cement are disproportionately developed, or that one of them is defective in its parts? Another and perhaps the most frequent predisposing cause of caries of the neck of the grinder teeth is that food becomes impacted between them. Its decomposition may not only affect the teeth, but the alveolar processes also."

The professor believes that caries of the crown of a tooth is generally caused by the horse biting on a stone or piece of metal during mastication. If the stone is lodged in the cavity of the infundibulum, the pulp of the tooth may be injured, for, to use the professor's words, "the thickness of the tooth between the upper part of the pulp-cavity and the bottom of the deepest infundibula is not very great."

Of the treatment of caries of the necks and crowns of grinder teeth, the professor says:

"As I am not aware of any treatment by which the decaying process can be stopped, I would as an experiment in suitable cases—that is, in those in which the diseased part may be got at—plug the tooth with gutta-percha, having first thoroughly cleaned the cavity. If the plug can be retained in its place, some benefit may be derived from its use. Believing, however, that the decomposition of food impacted between the grinder teeth is one of the exciting causes of their decay, I would advise that it be now and then removed. It would not only prevent decay, but in cases where decay had already begun, would to some extent check its progress. Indeed, I think the health of the horse would in many cases be improved by the adoption of such a plan."

While the professor recommends gutta-percha plugs for the crowns of slightly decayed grinders, he says that, compared with those of the necks, they are "less likely to be of even a slight benefit, inasmuch as the plug would be removed by attrition." Where the interior of the grinder is destroyed by disease, and the usual longitudinal fracture has occurred, he extracts the tooth with the forceps. While, as a rule, the tooth fractures longitudinally, the corners, he says, are sometimes broken off.

In commenting on the diseases of the alveolar processes, Prof. Varnell says:

"The causes which give rise to this condition of the maxillary bones are not easy to define. That a horse so affected is from certain peculiarities predisposed to it, there can be no doubt. For example, the teeth being placed at a distance from each other, thereby allowing the food to lodge between them, must be looked upon as a predisposing cause. A strumous diathesis, which I believe to be more common in the horse than is usually supposed, must also be regarded as a predisposing cause. The particles of food which become impacted in these unusually wide interdental spaces, after a time decompose and give rise to fetid compounds, which act prejudicially on the parts they are in contact with. The membrane which covers the gums, and also that which lines the alveoli and is reflected on the roots of the teeth, becomes inflamed. The inflammation will extend to the bone, the blood-vessels of which will become enlarged, as will also the Haversian canals in which they ramify. The osseous laminæ surrounding these canals will be partially absorbed, and to some extent separated from each other, and the enlarged spaces thus produced will be filled with inflammatory exudation. Hence the soft, spongy state of the gums and their tendency to bleed from slight causes; hence also the looseness of the teeth in the alveoli."

Of the deformity called *Parrot-Mouth*, and irregularities of the incisor teeth, Prof. Varnell says:

"This deformity consists in the upper incisor teeth projecting in front of and overhanging the lower ones to the extent in some instances of an inch and a half. The deformity resembles the upper bill of the parrot, which projects over the lower; hence the name. The lower incisors, from not being worn off by attrition, may become so long that the roof of the mouth is seriously injured. The deformity is generally associated with an irregular position of the upper grinders relatively with the lower.

"Sometimes the horse, when at pasture, is unable to take a sufficient quantity of food to keep himself in condition, and consequently he is considered legally unsound. But if fed from the manger he experiences little trouble in collecting his food; nor will his ability to masticate it be interfered with, except perhaps in old age.

"*Treatment.*—The treatment can only be palliative. If the roof of the mouth should become diseased and mastication impaired, the only remedy is to reduce the length of the lower incisors. The instrument generally used is a file or a rasp, but the process is so tedious and slow that it is seldom that much good is done. If the sliding-chisel could be brought to bear on them, their length could be readily reduced. Talking on the subject with my friend, Surgeon Gowing, he suggested a modification of this instrument which, I think, would answer very well.

"Irregularities of the incisor teeth, both with reference to their position and number, are even more common than in the grinders, but they seldom cause actual disease."

Prof. William Williams, like Prof. Varnell, has performed his part in elucidating the subject of caries of the teeth, and he has also illustrated the transmission of vitality to them from the outside—through the medium of the cement—after it has ceased to flow through the pulp on the inside, the pulp having become converted into dentine. It appears that anything that disturbs the equilibrium of this flow of vitality, which is the secret of the growth of the teeth throughout life, may cause caries. Prof. Williams says ("Principles and Practice of Veterinary Surgery," p. 470):

"Caries, dental gangrene, or decay, is almost exclusively confined to the grinder teeth—although I have seen the incisors in that condition—and may begin primarily in the root, neck, or crown of the tooth.

"Caries of the root arises from inflammation of the pulp, and may be caused by a constitutional predisposition or external injury. Inflammation of the pulp, however, does not always cause caries. I have several cases on record where the roots were enlarged from periodontal deposit, with abscesses surrounding the roots, without caries. Caries beginning at the roots may be due to the obliteration of the pulp-cavity at an age when the vitality of the tooth depends upon the integrity of the pulp. I need scarcely remind the professional reader that the integrity of the teeth depends upon a due supply, both as to quantity and quality, of nutritive materials.

"On the roots of a recently cut tooth but little cement is met with compared with that which exists in old teeth. As age advances the cement increases, and the tooth grows from the outside. In man it is generally agreed that after a given time the dentine ceases to be produced, and that the pulp is converted into osteodentine. In the horse the pulp-cavity becomes obliterated gradually by the pulp continuing to form dentine, the pulp simply giving way to its own product, which ultimately occupies its place and fills its cavity. In proportion as the pulp diminishes the supply of nutriment is lessened, until at length it is entirely cut off from the interior; to provide for the vitality of the tooth the cement increases in quantity on the root, and at the expense of the perfectly formed dentine lying in immediate contact with its inner surface. That is to say, this layer of dentine is converted into cement by the dentinal lacunæ undergoing dilatation and becoming identical with the hollow spaces or cells of the cement. The tooth now draws its nourishment from the blood-vessels of the socket, and thus continues, long after the obliteration of its pulp-cavity, to perform its part in the living organism.

"This is the natural condition of old teeth. But when the pulp-cavity is obliterated at an early age, by a too rapid formation of dentine, and consequent obliteration of the pulp when the cement is not yet sufficiently developed to supply nourishment to the whole tooth, caries must be the result. Many cases of caries that have come under my observation have resulted from this cause, and very often the disease is confined to that part of the cement that dips with the enamel into the interior of the tooth, splitting it into several longitudinal fragments.

"Caries of the neck of the tooth is seen in those horses whose teeth are wide apart, and is caused by the food remaining in the interspaces, and by decomposition exciting inflammation in the periodontal membrane. Caries of the neck is very commonly met with in the teeth of dogs, sometimes causing abscesses in the cheek.

"Caries beginning at the crown is due to a portion of the dentine losing vitality and the power of resisting the chemical action of the fluids of the mouth. A portion of the enamel of the crown may be fractured by biting a stone or piece of metal contained in the food. Mere fracture of the enamel, however, is insufficient of itself to lead to caries of the teeth in the lower animals, for it is a substance that is gradually worn off by mastication; but the violence which has caused fracture of the enamel, may at the same time have caused such an amount of injury to the dentine that it dies, and progressively becomes decomposed. In man it seems there should be death of the dentine and acidity of the oral fluids before caries can take place, test-paper applied to a carious tooth invariably showing the presence of free acid, and a very small perforation in the enamel may coexist with a considerable amount of disease in the dentine."

Surgeon T. W. Gowing, of London, a well-known inventor of dental instruments (veterinary), in an "Essay on the Diseases of the Teeth of the Horse," which was printed in "The Veterinarian" for 1851 (p. 632), in substance says:

"I am aware that the cause of disease of the teeth must to a certain extent always remain a mystery; yet from observation and reflection we may be able to deduce conclusions which practice will confirm.

"Let us consider the two classes of horses that we are principally called upon to attend, namely, the cart or draft-horse, and the hack or carriage-horse. So far as my observations have led me, the latter class are less liable to diseases of the teeth than those of a coarser breed. Now, may not this be caused by the better care they receive in the stable? The good and efficient groom regularly sifts the provender previous to feeding his horses, and thus rids it of stones, glass, &c. The cart-horse and the machine-horse of our London omnibus proprietors, not receiving this attention, are more subject to diseases of the teeth. Besides, it is a common practice with carters to sprinkle the provender with sulphuric acid, and we well know how acids affect the teeth. If such practices be allowed, diseases of the teeth may be readily accounted for.

"The teeth being lowly organized, soon lose their power of self-preservation. They are affected by the general health of the animal. Should the function of the stomach or alimentary track be deranged, the teeth—from the general health of the animal being interfered with, and from the local functional derangement—of all parts of the body, are the first to suffer or decay. Absorption of the gums, which may be caused by the decayed food that lodges between the grinders, is often followed by decay of the cement, which, being the most exterior as well as the most highly organized of the three substances composing the teeth, is the first to yield."

After describing the usual symptoms of diseased teeth, Surgeon Gowing asks:

"Who that has observed these symptoms, can hesitate for a moment to acknowledge that the animal is suffering pain, which, if we were to say arose from toothache, would not be believed by our employers?"

Prof. W. Youatt says in substance ("The Horse," p. 230):

"Of the diseases of the teeth we know little. Carious teeth are occasionally seen. They not only render mastication difficult, but they sometimes impart a fetid odor to the food, and the horse acquires a distaste for aliment altogether. Carious teeth should be extracted as soon as their real state is known, for the disease is often communicated to the contiguous teeth and to the jaw also. Dreadful cases of 'fungus hæmatodes' have arisen from the irritation of caries.

"Every horse that gets thin or out of condition, without fever or other apparent cause, should have his teeth and mouth examined, especially if, without any indication of sore throat, he 'quids' his food; or if he holds his head to one side while he eats, in order to get the food between the outer edges of his teeth. The cause is irregular teeth. Such a horse is materially lessened in value and is to all intents and purposes unsound, for although the teeth may be carefully sawn down, they will project again at no great length of time. A horse cannot be in full possession of his natural powers without perfect nutrition, and nutrition is rendered imperfect by any defect in mastication."

Prof. R. Owen, in his work entitled "A History of British Fossil Mammals and Birds" (pp. 388–9), gives an account of a diseased fossil horse's tooth which he found at Cromer. He says he is "induced to cite one of the curious examples of disease in an extinct animal from the rarity of its occurrence in the tissue which is the subject of it." The facts of this rare case are as follows:

"One of the Cromer fossil teeth, from the lower jaw, with a grinding surface measuring one inch five lines in long (antero-posterior) diameter, and eight lines in short (transverse) diameter, presented a swelling of one lobe, near the base of the implanted part of the tooth. To ascertain the nature and cause of this enlargement, I divided it transversely, and exposed a nearly spherical cavity, large enough to contain a pistol-ball, with a smooth inner surface. The parietes of this cavity, composed of dentine and enamel of the natural structure, were from one to two lines and a half thick, and were entire and imperforate. The water percolating the stratum in which this tooth had lain, had found access to the cavity through the porous texture of its walls, and had deposited on its interior a thin ferruginous crust; but the cavity had evidently been the result of some inflammatory and ulcerative process in the original formative pulp of the tooth, very analogous to the disease called 'spina ventosa' in bone."

## CHAPTER IX.

#### THE DENTISTRY OF THE TEETH.

Reports of Cases Treated by Various Surgeons.—Gutta-Percha as a Filling for Trephined Sinuses.—Teeth Pressing against the Palate.—Passing a Probe through a Decayed Tooth.—Death of a Horse from Swallowing a Diseased Tooth.

HORSEMEN, farmers, and other practical men will find much useful information in the present chapter, for it is based on the experiences of Veterinary Surgeons, whose reports appear in the various volumes of "The Veterinarian" (printed monthly in London), and to which I am so much indebted for other useful information. It is probably not too much to say that the more generally the chapter is read the fewer horses will be killed in the future for having decayed teeth, accompanied with a discharge from the nostril.

In "The Veterinarian" for 1856 (p. 437) Surgeon J. Horsburgh reports the following interesting case, entitled "Chronic Nasal Gleet produced by a Diseased Tooth:"

"About twelve months ago I was consulted about the case of a mare with a discharge from the near nostril. She had been under treatment for eighteen months, and the superior maxillary sinus had been opened with the trephine. The discharge, however, continued to flow, both from the nostril and the wound, notwithstanding the trephining had been performed a year before I saw the animal.

"The defluction had an offensive smell, and the submaxillary gland was enlarged, causing suspicion of glanders. The opening had been made a little too high, so that the central instead of the superior part of the sinus was perforated. I found that the whole mischief was caused by a diseased tooth. With the assistance of a smith I removed the tooth, which was split up its middle and considerably decayed. It was more than two inches long, and was bent forward toward the cheek. The odor was most offensive. I then opened the frontal and maxillary sinuses, both of which were filled with fetid pus. The wounds were first treated with a weak solution of chloride of lime, and subsequently with an ordinary astringent lotion. In addition to the local treatment, I administered the diniodide of copper.

"After a considerable time the wounds were allowed to heal, and the mare appeared much better. But very shortly the discharge began to flow again worse than ever, and the smell was almost intolerable. Determined, if possible, to make a cure of the case, I cut into the sinus again with the skull-saw, taking out a triangular piece of bone about two inches long by one inch and a half broad. At the upper part of the cavity I found some masticated food in a state of decomposition. It had passed through the alveolus into the sinus. Fractured bones were removed, and the opening being extended through into the nostril, a small instrument could be passed down it into the mouth. A weak nitric acid lotion was used to induce fresh inflammatory action, and, if possible, to fill up, by an effusion of lymph, the passage through which the food was pressed upward from the mouth into the cavity. The external wound was dressed with an ordinary healing lotion, and tow was put into it daily, and pressed downward to the mouth. A little blister liniment was also occasionally applied.

"Before operating, the frontal sinus on the affected side was considerably more bulging than the other. It is now reduced, and the wound has healed. The discharge from the nose has stopped, and there is no smell. Thus, after about two years and a half of treatment, this mare, now only five years old, is able to resume her work, and has every appearance of being likely to remain well.

"Had I not been able to effect a cure by the closing of the passage into the mouth, I would have tried filling it with gutta-percha. If a discharge were to take place again in this case, it would no doubt depend on the existence of a small aperture, and, under such circumstances, I should not hesitate to again cut into the sinus and endeavor to close the opening in the bone with gutta-percha, or some similar substance."

Surgeon H. Surmon, in an article "On the Extraction of Projecting Teeth," tells how he saved a horse that had been ordered killed by its owner ("Veterinarian," vol. ii, p. 25):

"Last year a neighbor of mine had a horse which had been losing flesh for some time, and his appetite was gradually diminishing. When I first examined the horse I saw no appearance of disease that could affect his appetite, and looking at his mouth I perceived no laceration of the cheeks or other injury. The horse grew worse, became almost a skeleton, and its owner ordered that it be killed. Being informed of the fact, I expressed a wish to examine his mouth once more. I accordingly put a balling-iron into his mouth and introduced my hand, and at the extremity of the grinders I found two teeth, one on each side of the lower jaw, which had grown long enough to press into the roof of the mouth, and thus prevented the animal from eating. I endeavored to extract these teeth with an instrument similar to that used for the human teeth, but without effect, as it could not be got on them. I then contrived an instrument which was very simple. When it was passed up the mouth, the tooth became fixed between the divided end of the iron; the handle being then turned, the tooth was extracted with the greatest ease. From that moment the horse began to feed, and rapidly improved in condition. In a short time he went to work, and has done well."

Surgeon C. May, of Malden, Eng., thus tells how he cured "A Case of Disease of the Jaw" ("Veterinarian," 1834, p. 93):

"I was requested by Mr. Ram, of Purleigh, to look at a horse which he told me had a 'cancer' in his jaw. I found my patient, a fine young chaise-horse, looking very poor, and having a constant discharge from the region of the root of the second lower grinder. There was considerable enlargement of the bone, which led me to suspect disease of the tooth, and which, on examination, proved to be true. On introducing a probe into the orifice, I found that it went through the tooth into the mouth. I was informed that this supposed cancer had been under the treatment of a farrier, and that the poor beast had been subjected to many painful caustic applications. As I was satisfied that no good could be done to the jaw as long as the tooth remained in it, I decided to extract it. I had an instrument made similar to the key used in human dentistry, with a handle like that of an auger. Having cast my patient and lanced the gum, I fixed the instrument on the tooth and succeeded in extracting it, although it required nearly all my strength. There was but trifling hemorrhage, and the 'cancer' soon got well. I think our patients are more frequently the subjects of toothache than we suppose. Perhaps 'quidding' in many of them might be traced to a carious tooth."

In a report of ten cases of diseased teeth that were treated at the Edinburgh Veterinary College during the year 1845, the details of one is thus given in "The Veterinarian" (1845, p. 626):

"A cart-horse was brought here with a profuse flow of white, clotty, and offensively smelling matter from the off nostril. The external plate of the superior maxillary bone on the same side was considerably elevated, and pain was evinced on pressing the part. There was no ulceration visible of the Schneiderian membrane, but the submaxillary lymphatic glands were somewhat enlarged. On examination there appeared to be disease of the superior maxilla, in which the grinder teeth were involved. Considering the extent to which the facial bones were affected, it was decided, as the only way of effecting a permanent cure, to extract the diseased teeth. The horse was cast, and by means of the ordinary tooth-key three of the upper back teeth were extracted. In a few days after the operation the discharge diminished in quantity, and under the continued application of proper remedies it entirely subsided, and the horse is now well.

"There are in this, as in former reports, cases where the superior maxillary bone and its sinuses have been injured from the elongation of the grinders of the inferior maxilla, causing a nasal discharge in many cases mistaken for that of glanders. They are easily remedied by shortening the teeth with the cutting-forceps."

Surgeon A. H. Santy says ("Veterinarian," 1875, p. 835):

"On the 26th of June I bought a six-year-old mare. She continued to work till July 17th, when she was suddenly taken with a slight running from the near nostril, which greatly increased in twenty-four hours. The submaxillary gland on that side swelled. There was slight tenderness of the throat and loss of appetite, which soon passed away. I showed the animal to a brother surgeon, and told him I thought of trephining. He said: 'Don't be in a hurry.' It struck me there might be something wrong with the grinders. I examined them, and found the fourth superior near side tooth with a depression on the outside and slightly raised from the surface of the other teeth. There was slight fetor from the food lodging there. I at once cast the mare, and with some difficulty extracted the tooth. I then dressed the wound and nursed the mare for a few days. The discharge from the nostril ceased in ten days. I have the mare now in constant work."

The above case deserves consideration for several reasons. Thousands of horses with precisely the same symptoms have been killed because the surgeon could not discriminate between diseased teeth and glanders. The "slight tenderness of the throat and loss of appetite, which soon passed away," was the result of the pus finding an outlet, which gave partial relief. Surgeon Sauty acted on the advice, "Don't be in a hurry," and consequently had time to think. The depression on the outside of the tooth and its slight projection above the common level, were signs that the trained eye only will detect. However, had the operation been delayed for a short time, in addition to the depression on the outside of the tooth, the gum would have been more or less shrunken, and the tooth, as a natural consequence, would have appeared longer.* Further, instead of the tooth being "slightly raised from the surface," it might have been below it; for, the inflammation having subsided, and the roots being shortened by the caries, it is liable to be forced deeper into the socket. Its next natural movement, the caries having destroyed its periosteum, is to drop out altogether.

As an offset to the foregoing cures, a few cases that terminated in death will be given. Surgeon Samuel Baker, in a letter to the editor of "The Veterinarian" (1845, p. 216), says:

"I was called in by a neighboring farmer to examine a two-year-old colt, which had to all appearance a polypus as large as a cricket-ball growing out of the right nostril. Respiration through that nostril was stopped. In order to ascertain its nature, I had the colt cast, and found that the nostril was filled with a hard fleshy tumor, which distended the other nostril also. After making an incision through the ala and side of the nostril, I removed a portion of the tumor, over a pound in weight. But, as still no air passed through, and

---

\* Shrinkage of the gum, according to C. D. House, invariably follows caries of the roots of the teeth.

there seemed not the slightest chance of gaining a passage, I ordered the colt to be killed.

"In dissecting the head I found that the cause proceeded from a decayed tooth, at the root of which was a bag of matter about the size of a walnut, which by no possible means could relieve itself."

Surgeon Baker does not say which of the six teeth (of course it was an upper grinder of the right side) was diseased. The complications of the case appear to have been unusual, otherwise the bag of matter would have sooner or later found an outlet through the nostril. The extraction of the tooth would have probably afforded an outlet through the alveolus; this failing, the effect of trephining the sinuses should have been tried.

Surgeon William Smith, of Norwich, Eng., reports a case of caries of the roots of several grinder teeth, accompanied by a discharge from the nostril, which he admits he mistook for ozena. He says ("Veterinarian," 1850, pp. 381–2):

"I was requested a few days ago to visit a horse which was supposed to be 'glandered.' I found the animal in a most emaciated and pitiable condition, with a copious greenish and very offensive discharge from the left nostril, with slight tumefaction of the gland on the same side. There was no appearance of ulceration, but the Schneiderian membrane had a leaden, dirty hue. Taking all the circumstances into consideration, I ordered the animal's destruction, but had its head sent to my infirmary.

"Meeting Surgeon Gloag, of the Eleventh Hussars, I told him I thought I had a case of ozena. He expressed a wish to be present at the examination of the head, and I was glad to avail myself of his assistance.

"A longitudinal cut was made on each side of the septum nasi, and a transverse one at a line between the center of the orbits. Another longitudinal cut, dividing the maxillary sinuses, was made just above the roots of the grinder teeth on each side. By this means we had an opportunity of examining the septum nasi on each side; also the turbinated bones, and the frontal and maxillary sinuses.

"On the left side we found an accumulation of pultaceous food, covered with thick pus, completely filling the maxillary sinus, and extending to the turbinated bones. The frontal sinus contained an accumulation of inspissated (thickened) pus, the septum nasi was of a leaden hue, as also the membrane covering the turbinated bones, which was much inflamed and thickened, but there was no appearance of ulceration.

"The difficulty was to ascertain how the food got there. After careful search, it was very evident that it could not have passed through the nostril. We therefore gradually dislodged the food and matter, searching for the former's entrance, and at last found a hole in the alveolar space belonging to the last grinder, the root of which was completely gone, only a small portion of the crown itself remaining. The hole was sufficiently large to admit the little finger. The mystery was solved—the process of mastication had deposited the food in the sinus. The fourth grinder was absent, having been lost evidently from previous disease.

"On examining the right side of the head we found the turbinated bones and membranes covering the septum nasi comparatively healthy, but we discovered a cyst, about the size of a walnut, in the maxillary sinus. It contained limpid fluid, and occupied the space immediately over the root of the fourth grinder tooth, which was decayed and quite loose, and *below*\* the level of the other teeth. The teeth of the lower jaw appeared healthy."

Without further examination, Surgeon Smith sent the head to the editor of "The Veterinarian," who says:

"The mare (that being the sex according to the teeth) we should take to have been about twenty years old. Her incisors are sound, and so are the grinders of the lower jaw. But in the near (left) upper jaw, the second, fourth, and sixth teeth are in a state of progressive decay, and the same is true of the fourth tooth of the off side. The vacuity caused by the defective last grinder has opened a passage to the antrum, through which the food has passed, and thence into the near chamber of the nose, between the turbinated bones, where it was discharged through the nostril. This accounts for the irritation on this side of the head, for the suppurated and even ulcerated condition of the Schneiderian membrane, and for the suspicious discharges. It was evident enough that there was no glanders. The very circumstance of alimentary matter being discharged through the nostril was enough to prove the contrary."

Still another case of destroying a horse for what merely appeared to be glanders is recorded by Prof.

---

\* The italics are mine. Compare with comments on Surgeon Santy's case, page 181.

William Percivall in his work entitled "Hippopathology" (vol. ii, p. 237). He says:

"There are instances on record of carious teeth being productive of such evil consequences as to lead, through error, to a fatal termination. The following relation ought to operate on our minds as a warning in pronouncing judgment in cases of glanders, or at least in such as assume the semblance of glanders:

"A horse, the property of government, became a patient of Surgeon Cherry on account of a copious defluction of discolored and purulent matter from the near nostril, unaccompanied by submaxillary tumefaction, or by ulceration of the Schneiderian membrane. For two or three months the case was treated for glanders; but no improvement following, a consultation was deemed necessary, the result of which was the horse was shot.

"On examination of the head, the third upper left grinder proved to be carious, one-third of its root being already consumed and the remainder rotten. The formation of an abscess within its socket had loosened the tooth, and the matter flowing therefrom had established a passage into the contiguous chamber of the nose. The antrum was also in part obstructed by the deposition of osseous matter.

"This is a case which, but for the inquisitiveness of Surgeon Cherry, would have merged into that heterogeneous class of diseases passing under the appellation of *chronic glanders*.

"My father's museum contained several specimens of carious teeth. One was that of a grinder, the interior of which was black and rugged, from being eroded by ulceration, and the roots had from the same cause mouldered away. Two others presented brittle exostoses upon their sides, forming spacious cavities within and communicating with the contiguous teeth. One of them exhibited a perforation through which pus appeared to have issued. Both seemed to have been cases which had originated in internal injury."

Prof. George Varnell closes his series of papers "On Some of the Diseases Affecting the Facial Region of the Horse's Head" ("Veterinarian," 1867), by giving an account of a case of 'osteo-sarcoma,' the disease, in his opinion, being caused by carious teeth. The case illustrates the importance of veterinary dentistry admirably. He says:

"Further to illustrate varieties of the diseases of the sinuses, I will relate a case of osteo-sarcoma which came under my care in July, 1862. I found the horse had an offensive discharge from the left nostril. The face below the orbit was enlarged, and the eye slightly displaced in its cavity. I also found that the three last grinder teeth in the upper jaw of the affected side were quite loose in their sockets, from which a discharge of a highly fetid character issued. Percussion on the side of the face indicated extensive disease, and the enlargement readily yielded to pressure. As there was not the slightest prospect of a cure, I suggested that the animal be killed.

"*Post-mortem Examination.*—The outer walls of the sinuses, which were very thin, were first removed, disclosing a mass of disease the seat of which was opposite the roots of the fourth grinder tooth, which was carious. This abnormal growth occupied the maxillary, malar, lachrymal, and a portion of the frontal sinuses, and had also encroached upon the orbit to such an extent as to displace the eyeball. The outer surface of the diseased mass was soft in texture. It had a gelatinous appearance, and when pressed with the blade of the scalpel, a thin, watery fluid oozed from its surface. A section of it presented a grayish-red appearance, with lightish streaks of fibro-osseous matter diverging from its roots and extending irregularly through its entire substance. The facial bones themselves, in the region of the disease, had in some parts disappeared altogether, while in others the cancelli were much enlarged, their osseous partitions partially absorbed, and their interstices filled with a deposition of a fibro-cellular structure.

"Such is a brief outline of this malignant and incurable disease, which I have no doubt primarily arose from caries of the roots of the grinder teeth."

Prof. Renault, of Alfort, France, is the author of an interesting account of a very unusual case, namely, the swallowing of a diseased tooth by a horse, which appeared originally in the "Recueil de Médicine Vétérinaire" for 1836. It is an argument against casting horses for the purpose of extracting their teeth, for had the horse been in a standing position the accident would not have occurred. When a horse's head rests upon the occiput, the muzzle pointing upward, it is as natural—the tooth being free of the forceps as well as the socket—for it to drop into the throat as it is for water to run down hill. The full history of the case is as follows:

"A post-horse, seven years old, had not fed well, and had been losing flesh during about three weeks. On the 20th of November, 1835, I saw him for the first time. The postilion told me that within the last two days he had eaten with more difficulty and pain than before, and dropped almost the whole of the hay and corn from his mouth before it was perfectly masticated. He had also observed that during the mastication of his food the horse always inclined his head to the left side.

"On examining the mouth, I easily recognized the cause of this difficulty of mastication. The gum, at the second grinder of the right lower jaw, was swollen and ulcerated, both within and without. The least pressure on the gum at this spot inflicted great pain, and the animal also suffered when the crown of the tooth was touched. On that portion of the jawbone contiguous to the diseased tooth, was a considerable swelling, hot and painful, which the postilion told me had existed for about twelve days. It was increasing in size every day. The breath was only slightly fetid, and there was nothing to indicate caries of the tooth. I expressed the opinion that the caries, if it existed, was confined chiefly to the root of the tooth, and that the ulceration of the alveolar septa beneath, of which there was no doubt, rendered its extraction necessary.

"On the following day the horse was cast, and his mouth being kept open by the proper instrument, the key was applied to the tooth. It resisted my first effort to draw it, but, on the second trial, gave way with a peculiar sound, which made me suspect that it was broken. The instrument (gag) was then taken out of the mouth, in order that the tooth might escape, but, to my great surprise, no tooth could be seen, notwithstanding I carefully searched for it. It was now plain that the tooth had been swallowed. I then assured myself that the tooth had been entirely extracted, and as, during the operation, the frænulum of the tongue had been wounded, I deferred the cauterization of the alveolus till the following day.

"As to the swallowing of the tooth, I gave myself very little concern. I did not think that so small a body was likely to form any serious obstruction in the intestinal canal, or that its temporary sojourn in the large intestine could become at all dangerous; so I merely directed that the mouth be frequently washed with warm water, and forbade the use of hard food.

"29th. I again saw the horse, and no serious consequence had yet followed the operation. He ate barleymeal mash with appetite, and a small quantity of hay. Two hours afterward he was brought to the School. He was very uneasy, and his belly was enormously distended, the swelling being principally on the right side, where the resonance was considerable on percussion. The horse was continually endeavoring to expel something from the anus, and the straining was so great that I feared the rectum would protrude. The efforts were followed by small mucous dejections, mixed with portions of food. The mucous membrane was of a subdued red color. These symptoms had been preceded by swelling at the flanks; colicky pains had followed, but they had ceased, and nothing now remained except the enlargement of the belly and the incessant effort to expel the fæces. The artery was full, but the pulse was almost imperceptible; the extremities were cold and the mucous membranes of a red violet color. The nostrils were convulsively dilated, respiration difficult and accelerated, and the walk staggering; the skin was covered with sweat, and, in a word, the animal presented every symptom of immediate suffocation. On this account I immediately opened the jugular and abstracted about twelve pounds of blood. The patient was very considerably relieved. I then ordered all four legs to be well rubbed with essential oil of turpentine.

"There now appeared to me a connection between these symptoms and the swallowing of the tooth. But where was this tooth? Entangled in the pyloric orifice of the stomach? I could not perceive any symptom of gastric disease. Was it in the convolutions or the cæcal portions of the small intestines? How then could I explain the distention of the large intestines and the expulsive efforts, so violent and continued? It was more likely that the tooth was lodged either in the colon or the cæcum, or in the irregularities of the floating colon, and partially or entirely prevented the passage of the fæces. It was hard to believe that in the lapse of two days the tooth could have reached the further part of the intestines.

"Having determined on the nature of the disease, I was somewhat embarrassed to ascertain its precise seat. I attempted to introduce my hand into the rectum, but the circumvolutions of the bowels were so much distended with gas, and so completely filled the pelvis, and the mere introduction of my finger caused such violent efforts to expel the contents of the rectum, that I was forced to desist.

"In the meantime the swelling rapidly increased, and again threatened suffocation. I then determined to use the only means in my power to prevent this, namely, to puncture the cæcum. This was effected with the trocar used for hoove in sheep, and in an instant the swelling subsided, and the symptoms of suffocation disappeared. I was then enabled to introduce my hand into the rectum, but I could not discover the situation of the tooth. While exploring the rectum;

however, the 'canula' escaped from the cæcum. The swelling now began again, and increased with extraordinary rapidity. I was about to plunge the trocar into the intestines once more, when I perceived that all treatment was useless. The animal was in the agonies of death, and in a few moments it expired.

"The post-mortem examination took place immediately after death. I found in the heart and lungs all the lesions which usually accompany death by suffocation. The digestive canal was distended by gas. The stomach was half filled with barleymeal, but not a particle of it was found throughout the whole extent of the small intestines, nor was there the slightest trace of inflammation of the mucous coat. The cæcum contained a great quantity of blood-tinted fluid, but there was no lesion or redness on any part of its internal face to indicate the source of the blood. Probably it came from the wound made by the trocar.

"In the cavity of the cæcum, toward its point, we found the tooth; but, I repeat it, there was no inflammation of its mucous membrane. There was, however, a slight discoloration of the membrane toward the end of the colon; it was of a slate color, and was probably caused by the sulphuretted hydrogen gas.

"Are we to conclude that the death of the horse was caused by the tooth? However extraordinary such a conclusion may at first appear, I am very much inclined to believe that it affords the best explanation of the mystery. The horse had scarcely eaten for fifteen days. This long fast had produced a comparatively empty condition of the digestive canal and an augmentation of its irritability up to the moment of the operation. The quietness of the horse and his appetite and apparent health during the two days preceding his death, proved that the tooth passed without obstacle through the first part of the intestinal canal. Having arrived at the cæcum, however, which was almost empty, and lying for a greater or less time at the inferior part of its mucous coat, its hard and irregular surface produced irritation; and as the contractions of this intestine were not effectual to seize the tooth and return it to the beginning of the colon, the prolongation of the irritation might suspend the digestive function of this viscus, augment its secretions, and cause the continual effort to expel the fæces. Hence also arose the gaseous distention of the abdomen. As to the death of the horse, the tooth was only the indirect cause. The direct cause was suffocation, which was produced by the distention of the bowels."

Prof. Bouley and Surgeon Ferguson report two fatal cases of swallowing teeth that came under their own observation. "In the first," they say, "the horse succumbed in a tympanitic affection, accompanied by extreme pain, and death was produced by asphyxia." The second case, judging by the short description of it in "The Veterinarian" for 1844, is the identical case just described by Prof. Bouley's fellow-townsman, Prof. Renault. Messrs. Bouley and Ferguson further say:

"Such, however, is happily not always the result of swallowing a tooth or the fragment of a tooth; but even the possibility of such a result ought to make the surgeon cautious. Moreover, the swallowing of a tooth may cause serious consequences at some future time. We refer to the formation of those productions called 'intestinal calculi.' The tooth, on account of its being indigestible, acts as the nucleus for the future calculus, as indeed may any similar body, which fact has been demonstrated by Prof. Morton, of the London Veterinary College, in an excellent paper on 'The Formation of Calculus Concretions in the Horse.'"*

Surgeon W. A. Cartwright reports that he extracted three grinders from a 'quidding' mare, one of which she swallowed ("Veterinarian," vol. iii, second series, p. 277). The tooth was sound, which may account for the favorable result of the case.

* *The Enterprise*, published in Virginia, Nevada, in its issue for December 12, 1878, contains an article entitled "A Stone found in a Horse's Jaw," which is in substance as follows: " For a long time a lump has been noticed in the side of the jaw of a horse belonging to Superintendent Osbiston, of the Gould and Curry and Best and Belcher mines. It was near the jawbone, and no liniment had power to soften or drive it away. Yesterday a veterinary surgeon made an incision, and to his astonishment removed a stone about two inches long and one inch in diameter. It is yellowish-white in color, and apparently as hard as marble. Mr. M. M. Frederick, the jeweler, divided it longitudinally, and in its center was what appeared to be a petrified grain of barley, which was also divided longitudinally. Around this nucleus the stone had formed in regular layers, the rings of which could be distinctly traced. The material of which the stone was composed appeared to be the same as that of the incrustations on the tubes of boilers. It is conjectured that the grain of barley pierced the gum and imbedded itself in the flesh, and that the saliva, flowing in, deposited limy matter similar to that which is sometimes found on the teeth of horses as well as men. A small concretion having thus been formed, it gradually grew, the channel by which the grain of barley entered no doubt remaining open and allowing an inflow of saliva."

The above case is another proof that Dr. Dunglison was right when he said that calculi "may form in every part of the animal body."

# CHAPTER X.

## FRACTURED JAWS.

How Caused, and how to Distinguish an Abrasion of the Gums from a Fracture of the Bone.—Replacing an Eye, Amputating part of a Lower Jaw, taking a Fractured Tooth and Bones out through the Nostril, &c.

FRACTURES of the jaws of the horse are of common occurrence. They may exist independently, but they are often complicated with and the cause of diseases of the teeth. Caries of the jawbone proper, and even some of the facial bones, is often communicated to the alveoli, and when necrosis ensues the destruction of the teeth is inevitable. This is as true in the case of the horse as in that of man.

The rami (branches) of the lower jaw are common seats of fracture, a frequent cause of which is the use of sharp curved bits; but rough usage by the rider or driver will now and then cause fractures even with a smooth bit. As a rule, at first, the gums only are affected; but in a short time the periosteum and bone are reached. Prof. Varnell says: "If the matter that escapes be of a grayish-brown color and fetid, it will indicate disease of the bone; but if it is from a subcutaneous abscess, the discharge will be simply of a purulent nature, and a speedy cure may be effected by the application of very simple remedies."

When a fracture has been produced, inflammation and fetor will follow, and the horse loses his appetite. If the bone is removed and the horse is allowed to rest for a few days, the wound will heal; otherwise the most serious consequences may follow. The removal of the bone may be effected sometimes soon after the fracture; but if, after cutting into the gum, it be found too firmly attached to the surrounding parts, it is better to wait a week or two that nature may loosen it. Bones an inch or more in length are often removed. Thus that which at first appears to be "only a sore mouth," may, if neglected, prove the ruin of a valuable horse.

Fractures are often caused by external violence. A severe blow, accidental or otherwise, in the region of the roots of the teeth may cause a fracture that will necessitate the removal of both the bone and the teeth.

"The lower jaw," says Prof. Youatt, "is more subject to fracture than the upper, particularly at the point between the tushes and the incisor teeth, and at the symphysis (of the chin) between the two branches of the jaw. Its position, length, and the small quantity of muscle covering it, especially anteriorly, render it liable to fracture. The same circumstances, however, combine to render a reunion of the parts easy."

The following extraordinary case of accidental fracture is reported by Surgeon George Fleming ("Veterinarian," 1874, p. 694):

"In 1865, while stationed near Aldershot, I was driving one day in the neighborhood of Farnborough, when, in a narrow lane, our progress was somewhat checked by a farmer's wagon in front, which compelled us to travel at a walking pace for some distance. During this delay my attention was attracted to the shaft horse, which had an enormous tumor on the right side of its face. It had such a singular appearance that I dismounted from the carriage and induced the driver of the wagon to halt, when I inquired into the history of the case, and made an inspection of the tumor. It was as large as half a good-sized cocoanut, occupied nearly the whole side of the face, and was literally a mass of what at first appeared to be fragments of bone, but which, on a closer examination, proved to be imperfectly developed grinder teeth. The tumor looked as if it were composed entirely of them. I was informed that, when two years old, the foal had taken fright and ran away, and in trying to get through a gate, a wooden stump ran into its face, making a large hole. The hole filled up, the tumor gradually formed on it, and since that time these 'bits of bone,' as the wagoner called them, were constantly shed from its surface. The growth was so large that the collar was passed over the head with great difficulty. I was so much interested in the case that I offered to keep the animal while the removal of the tumor was attempted; but the farmer could not spare it from work at the time, and I did not have another opportunity."

The following accounts of cases of fractured jaws treated by various surgeons are from Prof. Youatt's work, "The Horse" (p. 445):

"Surgeon Cartwright had a mare in which the upper jawbone was fractured by a kick at the point where it unites with the lachrymal and malar bones. He applied the trephine, and removed many small bones. The wound was then covered by adhesive plaster, and in a month the parts were healed.

"Surgeon Clayworth reports the case of a mare that fell while being ridden almost at full speed, and fractured the upper jaw three inches above the corner incisors. The teeth and jaw were turned, like a hook, completely within the lower teeth. The mare was cast, a balling-iron put into her mouth, and the teeth and jaw pulled back to their natural position; she was then tied so that she could not rub her muzzle against anything, and was fed with bean-meal and linseed tea. Much inflammation ensued, but it gradually subsided, and at the expiration of the sixth week the mouth was healed, scarcely a vestige of the fracture remaining.

"An account of a very extraordinary fracture of the superior maxillary bone is given in the records of the Royal and Central Society of Agriculture in France. A horse was kicked by another horse, fracturing the upper part of the superior maxillary and zygomatic bones, and almost forcing the eye out of its socket. Few men would have dared to undertake a case like this, but Monsieur Revel shrank not from his duty. He removed several small bones, replaced the larger ones, returned the eye to its socket, confined the parts with sutures, slung the horse, and in six weeks he was well.

"Surgeon Blaine relates that in treating a fracture of the lower jaw he succeeded by incasing the entire jaw in a strong leather frame. I have myself effected the same object by similar means.

"Prof. Bouley says ("Recueil de Médicine Vétérinaire," 1838) that he treated a horse whose lower jaw had been completely broken off at the neck—that is, at the point between the tushes and the corner incisor teeth, the detached bone being held by the membrane of the mouth.

"The horse was cast, the corner tooth on the left side extracted, the wound thoroughly cleansed, and the fractured bones brought in contact. Holes were drilled between the tushes and the second incisors of both jaws, through which brass wires were passed. A compress of tow and a ligature, the bearing-place of the latter being over the tushes, surrounded the whole. Thus the jaws were apparently fixed immovably together. The wires yielded somewhat to the struggles of the horse, but the bandage of tow was tightened so as to retain the fractured edges in apposition.

"The wound now began to exhale an infectious odor, and gangrene was evidently approaching. M. Bouley determined to amputate the fractured portion of the jaw, its union to the main bone being apparently impossible. The sphacelated portion of the jaw was entirely removed; every fragment of bone that had an oblique direction was sawn away, and the rough portions which the saw could not reach were rasped off.

"Before night the horse had recovered his natural spirits, and was reaching for something to eat. On the following day he ate oats, and no one looking at him would have suspected that he had been deprived of his lower incisor teeth. The next day he ate hay. In a fortnight the wound was nearly healed."

C. D. House, veterinary dentist, performed an unusual operation on a seven-year-old horse, the property of Mr. J. T. Allen, of Hartford, Conn. In 1876 a surgeon (?) made an incision in the right cheek and *knocked* out a large part of the fifth upper grinder. The violence of the operation fractured both the tooth and the jaw, imbedding a large fragment of the former in the bone above the socket. A year afterward, the horse still suffering and discharging matter from the nostril, Mr. House was requested by Mr. Allen to examine and if possible cure him. He failed, however, to discover the cause of the discharge, and it was not till the expiration of another year that he determined to probe the case to the bottom, the horse in the meantime having suffered as usual. Making an instrument of the proper size and shape, he introduced it into the nostril, seized the tooth fragment and drew it forth, the horse at that instant making a deep expiration, which blew out several fragments of bone and a part of the root of the tooth. The animal made a good recovery.*

* The Worcester, Mass., *Spy* for July 13, 1877, says: "C. D. House, veterinary dentist, was in the city yesterday, operating on the horses of the Hambletonian Breeding Stud. A case was found where the grinders had been worn rough, and were besides slightly displaced, so that the horse in eating lacerated the lining of the cheek. Another case was where a colt's temporary tooth, after being partially forced from its place by the permanent, had remained fastened by one root, and in such a position as to injure the gum while the animal was feeding; and yet so nicely had the decaying tooth been lodged, that its presence was only detected by the offensive odor. Several cases of inflammation of the gums were found, which were accounted for by the presence of tartar. The tartar was removed.

"Mr. House's mode of operating is unique. He uses no gag, and the animal stands free. He passes his hands over the teeth of the most vicious horses, and was never yet bitten. He has

---

Note.—In a paragraph of the above note that appeared in the first edition of this work, Dr. House, who now holds a diploma, advertised the importance of dentistry by depreciating the importance of that great scourge *glanders*, which Surgeon Fleming describes (1882) as a most repulsive, highly contagious, and incurable malady, very communicable between the horse and ass species, less so between these and other species, man also being frequently infected. Dr. Fleming says the disease was very prevalent in London in the winter of 1882.

Surgeon J. P. Heath thus describes a case of fractured jaw ("Veterinarian," 1878, p. 288):

"In May last I was called to see a horse that had been kicked by another horse. I found a transverse fracture of the left side of the lower jaw, between the first and second grinders, with lesion of the buccal membrane. The bone protruded inward, the tongue hung out of the mouth, and a constant flow of saliva existed. The animal's appetite was good, but there was of course a total inability to masticate. The horse was seventeen years old, but as the farmer (Mr. Gale, of Exminster, Devon,) could ill afford his loss, I agreed to try to cure him.

"I procured a wedge-shaped piece of wood, six or seven inches long by half an inch thick, which, after fitting it between the branches of the jaw, I well besmeared with warm pitch and pressed it tightly between the fractured end of the bone. I then fixed another piece of wood of the same length, but two inches thick, which was also besmeared with pitch, outside the fracture, placing a bandage six inches wide over the whole, and tying it over the face below the eyes.

operated on Edward Everett, Judge Fullerton, Emperor (owned by S. D. Houghton, of this city), and other notoriously vicious horses."

The statement about Mr. House's mode of operating is strictly true. His control of a horse appears to be a gift. He never confines a horse, not even in performing the operation of castration. In an "interview" with a reporter of *The New York Sun*, printed in 1877, in reply to the question, "How do you know when a horse has the toothache?" he said: "He *tells* me that he has it." So Mr. House must understand "horse-talk" as well as horse-dentistry.

"For the first fortnight I do not think the animal took more than a gallon of the thin mashes and gruel with which he was supplied; but after that time the use of the muscles of the tongue began to return, and he was able to swallow a little. In about three weeks he could lick up oatmeal and oilcake gruel made thick, and in less than a month I removed the bandage (although the splints remained for six weeks), as by this time he could swallow a little pulped mangold grass, cut into chaff. For nine weeks he could only feed on cut fodder, when he was turned out to grass. At the present time he is in perfect health, feeding on ordinary diet and working constantly. The first and second grinders, which were loosened, appear now to be as firmly fixed as the others."

The editor of "The Veterinarian" reports the case of a pony that came near starving from having a stick fastened in its mouth. No fracture of the bone was produced, but the account of the case is worthy of insertion here notwithstanding that fact, for it illustrates a class of mishaps to which the horse is subject. He says ("Veterinarian," 1855, p. 330):

"A pony was turned into a pasture, and was not seen for several days. The owner found it standing in a corner of the field, looking dejected and thin, with a small quantity of viscid saliva escaping from its mouth. He took care of the pony for a few days, during which time it took nothing but a little water, which it drank with great difficulty. Our attendance was now requested. Examination disclosed a stick about the size of one's finger, firmly wedged across the palate, between the corner incisors. Its pressure had produced extensive sloughing, so that the bone was completely exposed. The pain was so great that the poor animal stoutly resisted our efforts to remove the cause of its suffering. This, however, was soon done, and the parts being cleaned with tepid water, were afterward dressed with Tinct. Myrrhæ. Little after treatment was necessary beyond the daily application of the tincture, a mash diet, and the substitution of oatmeal gruel for plain water."

# CHAPTER XI.

### THE TEETH AS INDICATORS OF AGE.

Their various ways of Indicating Age.—The "Mark's" Twofold Use.—The Dentinal Star.—Marks with too much Cement.—Tricks of the Trade. —Crib-biting.—Signs of Age Independent of the Teeth.

The incisor teeth of the horse, which, as before said, differ "from those of all other animals by the fold of enamel which penetrates the body of the crown, from its broad, flat summit, like the inverted finger of a glove," indicate age (1) by their cutting; (2) by their growth; (3) by their shedding; (4) by their marks;* (5) by their change of shape; (6) by their change of color; (7) by their length, and (8) by the degree of their outward inclination. The cutting, growth, and shedding (of the tushes and grinders as well as the incisors—the cutting and shedding occurring at comparatively regular periods, and the growth being gradual), indicate age from birth till about the sixth year; the marks of the lower incisors from the sixth month till the eighth year; those of the upper incisors, though

---

* Prof. C. S. Tomes says "the mark exists in Hipparion, but not in the earlier progenitors of the horse." Prof. O. C. Marsh says: "The large canines of Orohippus became gradually reduced in the later genera, and the characteristic mark of the incisors is found only in the later forms."

perhaps less reliable, during the same period, and for about four or five years longer (say the twelfth or thirteenth), and the change in shape,* color, and position from about the seventh year till old age. The change in the shape of the teeth is caused by their wear and growth, the wear counteracting the growth and the growth the wear.

In foals and young horses the marks are probably the surest guides by which to judge of the age. One peculiarity of them is that, as the teeth wear down, they approach the posterior edge. Besides their utility in indicating age—being composed of enamel (the adamantine substance)—they greatly enhance the durability of the teeth—that is, during the first third of the horse's life. As a rule the variations in the size and appearance of the mark will be as follows:

At six months they are oblong and distinct in the centrals, and the cavities are plain in the dividers.

At one year they are short in the centrals, are becoming so in the dividers, but are large in the corners.

At a year and a half they are represented by a small spot in the centrals, are diminished in the dividers, but are still large in the corners.

At two years they are no longer visible in the centrals (in some cases are even shed); are smaller and rounder in the dividers, but still plain in the corners.

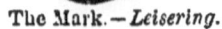
The Mark.—*Leisering.*

---

* Surg. Cherry says the shape and general character of the teeth are better criterions of age than the marks.

At two years and a half the centrals are shed; the marks are faint in the dividers, but are distinct in the corners.

At three years the permanent centrals are nearly grown; the marks in the dividers are just visible, and have become smaller in the corners.

At three years and a half the marks in the centrals are long and very distinct; the dividers are shed, and the marks in the corners are faint.

At four years the marks in the centrals show the effects of wear, but are still long and distinct; the permanent dividers are about grown, and the marks in the corner teeth have almost disappeared.

At four years and a half the marks in the centrals are still distinct, while those of the dividers are at their best. The contrast between the large permanent incisors and the small temporary corner teeth, which have lost their marks, is striking at this age.

At five years the marks in the centrals are getting smaller and rounder, but are large and distinct in the dividers; the corners are usually shed at this age.

"At six years," says Prof. Youatt, "the marks of the central nippers are worn out. There will, however, still be a difference of color in the center of the tooth. The cement filling the hole made by the dipping of the enamel will present a browner hue than the other part of the tooth. It will be distinctly surrounded by an edge of enamel, and there will remain even a little depression in the center, and also around the case of enamel; but the deep holes in the center of the teeth, with the blackened surface which they present, and also the elevated edge of enamel, will have disappeared. Persons little accustomed to horses are often puzzled here. They expect to find a plain surface of uniform color, and know not what conclusion to draw when they see both discoloration and irregularity." The marks in the dividers are much reduced in size, but those of the corner teeth are large and distinct.

At seven years the marks disappear from the divider incisors, and at eight from the corner teeth.

Monsieur Girard thus describes the changes in shape of the incisors, referring also to the disappearance of the marks in the upper teeth:

"At nine the central incisors become rounded, the dividers oval, and the corner teeth narrower. The central enamel (mark) diminishes and approaches the posterior edge.

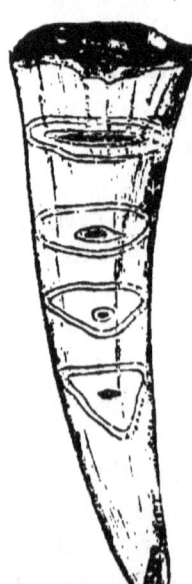

The forms successively assumed by the dental table of an incisor in consequence of friction.—*A. Chauveau.*

"At ten the dividers are rounder, and the central enamel is very near the posterior edge and rounded; at eleven they have become rounded, and the enamel has disappeared.

"At twelve the corner teeth are rounded. The yellow band is larger, and occupies the center of the wearing surface.

"At thirteen all the lower incisors are rounder; the sides of the centrals are becoming longer. The central enamel remains in the upper corner teeth, but is round and approaching the posterior edge.

"At fourteen the lower central incisors have a triangular appearance; the dividers are becoming long at their sides.

"At fifteen the central incisors are triangular, and the dividers are becoming so.

"At sixteen the dividers are triangular, and the corner teeth are becoming so.

"At seventeen the corner teeth, like the dividers and centrals, have become triangular, the sides of the triangles being equal.

"At eighteen the lateral portions of the triangles lengthen in succession—first in the centrals, next in the dividers, and then in the corners; so that at nineteen the lower centrals are flattened from one side to the other; at twenty the dividers are flattened, and at twenty-one the corners also are."

The three following extracts give some idea of the difficulties to be encountered in judging the age by the teeth. Prof. Youatt says:

"Stabled horses have the marks sooner worn out than those at grass, and a 'crib-biter' may deceive the best judge by one or two years. At eleven or twelve the lower nippers change their original upright position and project forward. They become of a yellow color, the cause of which is that the teeth grow to offset their wear; but the enamel which covered their surface when they were young cannot be repaired, and that which wears this yellow color in old age is the part which was formerly in the sockets. The gums recede and waste away, and the tushes wear to stumps and project outward."

Surgeon Ewd. Mayhew says ("The Horse's Mouth: Showing the Age by the Teeth"):

"That the teeth of the horse denote age appears to have been a very ancient belief, which the experience of centuries has not changed. Within certain limits the belief is well founded, for perhaps no development is more regular than the teeth of the horse, and no natural process so little exposed to the distortions of artifice. We are, nevertheless, not to expect that the animal carries in its mouth a certificate of birth, written in characters so deep that they cannot be obliterated or misinterpreted. He who would judge of the age by the teeth must study them, and be prepared to encounter difficulties. In proportion as he has done the one, and is enabled thereby to overcome the other, will be his success. The qualified judge alone will read the teeth correctly. He will make allowance where certain marks are indistinct or absent, and he will be cautious in pronouncing an opinion. The veterinary practitioner knows that the teeth are worthy of attention, and he feels that their indications, scientifically interpreted, will seldom mislead."

Surgeon J. H. Walsh, in his excellent work, "The Horse; in the Stable and in the Field," says:

"In order to be able to estimate the age of the horse by his teeth, it is necessary to ascertain, as nearly as may be, the exact time at which he puts up his milk teeth, and also the periods at which they were replaced by the permanent. Finally it becomes the province of the veterinarian to lay down rules for ascertaining the age from the degree of attrition which the permanent teeth have undergone. For these several purposes the horse's mouth must be studied from the earliest period of his life up to old age."

Judging the age by the teeth is even more complicated and difficult than is shown by the foregoing extracts. Among other complications worthy of consideration are the following:

About the ninth year a mark, which is sometimes mistaken for the infundibulum, appears on the central incisors. Girard named it the *dentinal\* star*, but it is also called the *fang-hole* and *secondary mark*. Dentinal star is perhaps the most proper name, for the mark is "due to the presence of secondary *dentine*, into which the remains of the pulp has been converted." The conversion of the pulp into dentine prevents 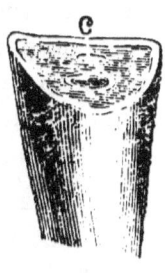 the cavity from becoming a reservoir for food, for otherwise it would become such as soon as reached by wear; and it preserves the tooth from decay, affording a good illustration of Nature barricading disease. The pulp cavity is lined with dentine; the dentine into which the pulp is converted is sometimes called osteodentine, and may be distinguished from the former by its yellow tint. The star may not afford reliable data by which to judge of the age, but its presence is *prima facie* evidence that the tooth has been worn to the original pulp cavity.† It becomes plainer as it approaches the cavity's center, but the bottom of the cavity is ultimately reached, which of course is hollow. It is visible 8 or 10 years, the depth of the cavities varying from about ⅜ to 1 inch.

The marks of some teeth are disproportionately composed of cement, a fact Prof. A. Chauveau says he is not aware has ever been taken into account in "cal-

---

\* See note, page viii.

† Nature fills the cavity in proportion as the crown is worn. Take two teeth of the same kind, one just full-grown, the other worn almost to its neck. In the latter the spot is visible, and if as much material is cut from the former as has been worn from the latter, its cavity will be cut through.—*John Hunter.*

culating the progress of wear." Such teeth would soon wear out, for there is as much difference in the density of cement and enamel as between cartilage and bone.

The obliteration of the mark may be hastened in a small or medium-sized tooth by the friction of one that is abnormally large, while a stunted or dead tooth may never lose its mark.

The more upright the teeth the faster they wear. It is said that the crowns will be worn to the extent of a quarter of an inch between the fifth and sixth years (when they are most upright), while only about that quantity of material will wear away between the twentieth and twenty-fifth years.

A horse's food is a matter also to be taken into account. The mastication of grass, carrots, turnips, potatoes, bread, &c., does not cause much wear to the teeth. However, when grass is procured by grazing the incisors suffer much friction—caused, not by the grass, but by the teeth grinding one another, for they meet edge to edge, and are employed in this occupation for hours, whereas a "feed" of corn is shelled in a few minutes. In the former case the incisors suffer great friction; in the latter, the grinders. Again, it is said that "horses fed on salt marshes, where the sea-sand is washed among the grass, or on sandy plains or meadows, are affected by the increased friction of their teeth." But no matter how soft a horse's food may be, if he is addicted to the vice called "crib-biting," his teeth may be ruined before those of the corn-fed horse have even lost their marks.

Several trade tricks are also to be noted. Of "bishoping," Prof. Youatt says:

"Dishonest dealers resort to a method of imitating

the mark in the lower nippers. It is called *Bishoping,* from the name of the scoundrel who invented it. The horse of eight or nine years is thrown, and with an engraver's tool a hole is dug in the now almost plain surface of the corner teeth, its shape resembling the mark in those of a seven-year-old horse. The hole is then burned with a heated iron, and a permanent black stain is left. The next pair of nippers are sometimes lightly touched also.

"An unprofessional man would be easily deceived by this fraud, but it cannot deceive the trained eye of the horseman. The irregular appearance of the cavity, the diffusion of the black stain around the tushes— the sharp points and concave inner surface of which can never be given again—the marks on the upper nippers, together with the general conformation of the horse, will prevent deception. Moreover, in comparing the lower with the upper nippers, unless the operator has performed on the latter also, they will be found to be considerably more worn than the lower, the reverse of which ought to be the case. Occasionally a clever operator will burn all the teeth to a properly regulated depth, and then a practiced eye alone will detect the imposition."*

---

* ROUGH ON THE RUSSIANS.—Surgeon John C. Knowlson makes the following open confession ("The Complete Farrier, or Horse Doctor," p. 150): "I was hired by Anthony Johnson, of Wincolmlee, Hull, as farrier to a number of horses that were going to Moscow, Russia. We had a little gray, seventeen-year-old horse, named *Peutum*, whose mouth I bishoped. He passed for six years old, was the first horse sold, and brought £500, English money! I only mention this as a caution to horsemen."

Surgeon Knowlson could have evidently beaten the late President Lincoln in a (wooden) horse trade.

Of a deception practiced by sellers of two-year-old foals, namely, passing off an early two-year-old for a late three-year-old, Prof. Youatt says:

"The age of all horses used to be reckoned from May, but some are foaled as early as January. A two-year-old foal of the latter date may, if it has been well nursed and fed and has had its central nippers drawn (that three or four months' time may be gained in the appearance of the permanent), be sold at the former date for a three-year-old. To horsemen, however, the general form of the animal, the little development of the forehand, the continuance of the mark in the divider nippers, its more evident existence in the corner ones, and some enlargement or irregularity about the gums, from the violence used in forcing out the teeth, are a sufficient security against deception."

And again of four-year-old foals:

"Now, more than at any other time, will the dealer be anxious to put an additional year upon the animal, for the difference in strength, utility, and value between a four-year-old colt and a five-year-old horse is very great. But the lack of wear in the central and divider nippers, the small size of the corner ones, the little growth of the tushes, the low forehand, the legginess of the colt, and the thickness and little depth of the mouth, will at once detect the cheat."

The following is Prof. Youatt's description of crib-biting and its effect on the teeth ("The Horse," pp. 511, 519):

"The horse lays hold of the manger with his teeth, violently extends his neck, and then, after some convulsive action of the throat, a slight grunting is heard, accompanied by a sucking in of air. It is not an effort at simple eructation, arising from indigestion, but is merely the inhalation of air. It takes place with all kinds of diet, and when the stomach is empty as well as when it is full.

"The effects of crib-biting are plain enough. The teeth are worn away and occasionally broken, and in old horses to a very serious degree. Sometimes grazing is rendered difficult or almost impossible. Corn is often wasted, for the horse will frequently 'crib' with his mouth full of it, and the greater part of it will fall over the edge of the manger. Much saliva escapes also, which impairs digestion. Crib-biting horses are more subject to colic than others, and to a species difficult of treatment and frequently dangerous.

"The only remedy is a muzzle, with bars across the bottom sufficiently wide to allow the horse to pick up his corn and pull his hay, but not to grasp the edge of the manger. Some recommend turning out for five or six months; but this will never succeed except with young horses, and rarely with them. The old crib-biter will substitute the gate for the manger. We have often seen him galloping across the field for the mere object of having a gripe at a rail."

Prof. Youatt further says that the vice is a species of unsoundness, having been so decided in the courts. It is often the result, he says, of imitation, but oftener the consequence of indigestion. Mischief, he says, is another cause of it.

The mouth, it is said, is broader at seven years of age than at any other time; but, so far as judging the age is concerned, this fact (assertion) is of little practical use. The facts that follow, however, are of more or less use, and are worthy of perusal. Prof. Youatt says:

"The indications of age, independent of the teeth, are deepening of the hollows over the eyes; wrinkles over the eyes and about the mouth; gray hairs, particularly over the eyes and about the muzzle; the countenance and general appearance; thinness and hanging down of the lips; sharpness of the withers; sinking of the back; lengthening of the quarters, and the disappearance of windgalls, spavins, and tumors of every kind. * * * At nine or ten the 'bars' of the mouth become less prominent, and their regular diminution will indicate increasing age."

Of another deception Prof. Youatt says:

"We form some idea of the age of the horse by the depth of the pits above the eyes. There is at the back of the eye a quantity of fatty substance, on which it may revolve without friction. In aged horses, and in diseases attended with general loss of condition, much of this disappears. The eye becomes sunken, and the pit above it deepens. Dishonest dealers puncture the skin, and, with a tobacco-pipe or tube, blow into the orifice till the depression is almost filled. This, with the aid of 'bishoped' teeth, may deceive the unwary. The fraud may be easily detected, however, by pressing on the part."

"Frank Forester" (William Henry Herbert), says ("The Horse of America," vol. i, p. 72):

"Much stress is laid by many persons on the depth of the supra-orbital cavities, and more yet on the length and extreme protrusion of the nippers beyond the gums, as also on hollowness of back. I have seen colts —*got by aged stallions*—having all these indications of age before they had a full mouth; and with cavities and hollow backs before they had got colt's teeth."

Surgeon Brandt, who thinks *shape* indicates age as well after the eighth year as marks do before, says (" Age of Horses "):— " Some breeds, the Spanish for instance, require a longer time to develop than others. The bones appear to be harder, the teeth change somewhat later, and wear more slowly; sometimes, after the fifth year, they appear one or two years younger than they are. The age of crib-biters can be told by the corner teeth, which are seldom injured. Should this be the case, how-

Pliny did not compile Varro (B. C. 116) and Columella (A. D. 42) carefully. Varro (Book II., Cap. VII.) says: "It is by the teeth that they find out the age of a horse." He then describes the shedding of the teeth, concluding as follows: "Others grow in their place, which, hollow at first, fill up in the sixth year," etc. The error about the cavities filling up stands to this day. Unlike the pulp cavities, they are not filled by nature with tooth material; they are obliterated by wear. Columella (Book VI., Cap. XXIX.) not only describes the marks, but the shedding of the molars also. In Latin he says: "*Intra sextum deinde annum, molares superiores cadunt.*" So the error of Aristotle about the non-shedding of the molars did not stand till the sixteenth century. (See page 69.) Palladius (about A. D. 400) and Vegetius (about the same time) describe both the marks and the shedding of the molars. Vegetius speaks of the wrinkles in the upper lip, the number of wrinkles indicating the

al use. The facts that follow, however, are of more
less use, and are worthy of perusal. Prof. Youatt
is:

"The indications of age, independent of the teeth,
 deepening of the hollows over the eyes; wrinkles
er the eyes and about the mouth; gray hairs, par-
ularly over the eyes and about the muzzle; the
untenance and general appearance; thinness and
nging down of the lips; sharpness of the withers;
aking of the back; lengthening of the quarters, and
number of years, and also the black spots in the middle of the teeth about the twelfth year. In conclusion he says: "Finally, the number of wrinkles, the sadness of the countenance, the stupor of the eyes, the baldness of the eyelids, the dejection of the neck, and the lassitude of the whole body indicate age." (Book IV., Cap. V.) I have never seen what could be called a description of the wrinkles in any other book, but my attention was called to them by Dr. Wm. Wilson, of Jersey City, N. J., in 1881. Vegetius Renatus, *Publius*, is often confounded with Vegetius Renatus, *Flavius*, a military author. Vegetius wrote on veterinary science; Varro, Columella and Palladius on agriculture. Fragments of the works of Apsyrtus (or Absyrtus), the Greek veterinarian (about A. D. 330), are extant, but I have never seen anything of his on age. He described glanders, fevers, epizootic influenza, dental cysts, etc. (See JOURNAL OF COMPARATIVE MEDICINE AND SURGERY for January, 1884, page 19.)

gums, as also on hollowness of back. I have seen colts —*got by aged stallions*—having all these indications of age before they had a full mouth; and with cavities and hollow backs before they had got colt's teeth."

Surgeon Brandt, who thinks *shape* indicates age as well after the eighth year as marks do before, says ("Age of Horses"):— "Some breeds, the Spanish for instance, require a longer time to develop than others. The bones appear to be harder, the teeth change somewhat later, and wear more slowly; sometimes, after the fifth year, they appear one or two years younger than they are. The age of crib-biters can be told by the corner teeth, which are seldom injured. Should this be the case, however, add as many lines as are needed to make them the natural length. The horse is as many years younger as the teeth are lines too short. The front teeth are frequently worn away earlier when horses have been fed on unshelled corn.

"The age of mules cannot be ascertained with the same accuracy as that of horses. After their eighth year they usually appear younger than they are."

*Note.*—C. F. Hoeing, M.R.C V.S. (Jersey City, N.J.) says the fact that the marks indicate age was discovered by Prof. Pessina of Vienna in 1818-20.

The ancients appear to have known nothing about the *marks*. Aristotle (His. Animals, Bohn's trans., pp. 170 1) says that before casting its teeth a horse has its mark, *but not afterward*. After casting them age is not easily told, but is usually ascertained by the canines, which in riding-horses are generally bit-worn; these teeth are called the *marking teeth*. (That is they are marked by wear. They have no *natural* marks. See p. 69.)

Xenophon, who finds use for tushes in bridling a horse—pressing the lip against them—says that in buying a horse, "to avoid being cheated, let it not escape notice what his age is; if he has not the foal teeth, he can neither give pleasure with anticipated exertion nor be easily disposed of." (p. 719.)

Pliny says age is indicated by the eruption and shedding of the incisors (giving accurate dates); then by the projecting of the teeth, the grayness of the eyebrows, and the depth of the pits around them. (Vol. iii. p. 60.)

Pliny compiled from Varro, Columella, and many others. Would they all fail to mention the marks if they knew anything about them?

*Erroneous and Extraordinary Statements by Pliny.*—Horses' teeth grow whiter with age. If a horse is gelded before it changes its teeth it never sheds them. No animal sheds the molars. Men have more teeth than women. All men, except the Turduli, have 32 teeth. Some persons have a continuous bone in place of teeth. Human teeth contain venom; they tarnish a mirror and kill unfledged pigeons. Zocles had a set of teeth at 104.

# CHAPTER XII.

## THE TRIGEMINUS OR FIFTH PAIR OF NERVES.

### Its Nature and the Relation it bears to the Teeth.—Its Course in the Horse and in Man.

THE thread-like nerves of the teeth are derived from the superior and inferior maxillary branches of the trigeminus or fifth pair of nerves. In the horse these branches are four or five times as thick as a ribbon and about five-eighths of an inch wide. The ophthalmic branch is smaller and shorter, its course extending only from the brain to the eye, while that of the two former extends to the lips, running parallel to and about an inch from the roots of the grinder teeth.*

The description of the trigeminus and its course is from a lecture by Prof. Youatt to veterinary students, and may be found in "The Veterinarian" for 1834 (p. 121). In the first part of the lecture the nature of the trigeminus—its double origin and function—is expatiated upon, a summary of which is that the sensitive and motor roots, are contained within the same sheath; that the sensitive root is so much larger and its fibrils so much more numerous than the motor that

---

* For the preparation of an anatomical specimen showing the general course of the trigeminus, I am indebted to Prof. J. M. Heard, of the New York College of Veterinary Surgeons.

it may still be called the sensitive nerve of the face; that the trigeminus is the only nerve of the brain that bestows sensibility to the face, except a few branches from the cervicals, which may be traced to the lower part of it; that there are some anatomical facts which incontestably prove that the motor nerve exists; that Sir Charles Bell laid the root of the trigeminus bare in an ass immediately after the animal's death, and that on irritating the nerve the muscles of the jaw acted and the jaw closed; that he divided the root of the nerve in a living animal, and the jaw fell;\* that he

---

\* "RE-ESTABLISHMENT OF SENSIBILITY AFTER RESECTION OF NERVES.—A memoir by MM. Arloing and Tripier was read before the French Academy, November 28th, on the effect of resection of certain nervous trunks. Clinical facts have several times shown that after wounds which have altered or destroyed a portion of a nerve, sensibility returns in the integuments to which the nerve is distributed. MM. Arloing and Tripier made nervous resections in dogs, and saw sensibility reappear after a certain time in the integuments to which the branches of the nerve were distributed, and in the peripheral end of the nerve itself."—*Popular Science Review, 1867.*

"HOW MOTOR-NERVES END IN NON-STRIATED MUSCULAR TISSUE.—A very valuable communication stating the results of M. Hénocque's researches has been published in "l'Archives de Physiologie," and may be thus abstracted: 1. The distribution of the nerves in smooth muscle is not only identical in man and other vertebrate animals in which it has been observed, but is essentially similar to all the organs containing smooth muscle. 2. Before terminating in the smooth muscle, the nerves form three distinct plexuses or networks—(*a*) a chief or fundamental plexus, containing numerous ganglia, and situated *outside* the smooth muscle; (*b*) an intermediate plexus; and (*c*) an intramuscular plexus, situated *within* the fasciculi of smooth fibers. 3. The terminal fibrils are everywhere identical. They divide and subdivide dichotomously, or anastomose, and terminate by a slight swelling or knob, or in a punctiform manner. The ter-

divided the superior maxillary branch on both sides, the animal losing the power of using the lips; that Mr. Mayo divided the root of both the superior and inferior maxillary, the result being that the lips no longer remained in perfect apposition, and the animal ceased to use them in taking up his food; that the sensitive root, or a portion of it, after entering the cavernous sinus, swells out into or passes through a ganglion, and that the motor root can be traced beyond the ganglion, uniting afterward with its fellow and forming the perfect nerve; that the ganglion, being composed of sensitive fibrils only, resembles a brain.

minal swelling appears to occupy different parts of the smooth muscular fiber, but most frequently to be in the neighborhood of the nucleus, or at the surface of the fibers, or, lastly, between them."—*The Monthly Microscopical Journal, 1870.*

"STRUCTURE OF NERVES.—M. Roudanoosky says that the primitive elements of nerves are tubes having a pentagonal or hexagonal configuration. As to their constitution, he says that every nerve has a substratum of brain-matter, and also of the spinal marrow, and probably of the ganglionic matter also. The gray matter, he says, is the fundamental nervous substance, and plays the principal part in the functions."—"*Veterinarian,*" *1865, p. 313.*

In a letter to his brother, G. J. Bell, written in 1807, Sir Charles says: "I consider the organs of the outward senses as forming a distinct class of nerves. I trace them to corresponding parts of the brain, totally distinct from the origin of the others. I take five tubercles within the brain as the internal senses. I trace the nerves of the nose, eye, ear, and tongue to these. Here I see established connection; there, the great mass of the brain receives processes from the central tubercles. Again, the great masses of the cerebrum send down processes or crura, which give off all the common nerves of voluntary motion. I establish thus a kind of circulation, as it were."—*Medical Gazette.*

Prof. Youatt's description of the course of the trigeminus is as follows:

"The trigeminus has been described as springing by a multitude of filaments from the crura cerebelli, and forthwith running for safety into the cavernous sinuses, and there suddenly enlarging into or passing through a ganglion. The nerve, as its name implies, divides into three parts, the division taking place in the cavernous sinus, after the superior or sensitive root has been joined by the inferior or motor root. Each part, before it leaves the cranium, assumes a distinct investment of dura mater. The branches are named, from the parts to which they are destined, the Ophthalmic, the Superior Maxillary, and the Inferior Maxillary.

"The *ophthalmic* is the smallest of the three. It is formed within the sinus, where it is in conjunction with the superior maxillary, which it soon leaves, and, passing through the foramen lacerum into the orbit, subdivides and forms three distinct branches—the Supra-orbital (the frontal), the Lachrymal, and the Lateral Nasal (the nasal). The supra-orbital climbs behind the muscles of the eye, giving filaments to the rectus superior and the superior oblique, and some also to the fatty matter of the eye. The main branch, escaping through the superciliary foramen, is soon lost in ramifications on the elevator of the superior eyelid, the integument of the forehead, and the periosteum. The lachrymal, as its name implies, is chiefly concerned with the lachrymal gland; a few ramifications, however, are sent to the conjunctiva and also to the ciliary glands of the upper eyelid, while a distinct twig of it passes out at the angle between the zygoma and the frontal orbital process, where it anastomoses with the supra-orbital and with ramifications from the superior maxillary. It is also lost on the integument and muscles of the forehead. The lateral nasal is the largest of the three. Almost at its beginning we observe the filaments that help to form the Ophthalmic Ganglion. They are more numerous and more easily traced in some of our domesticated animals than in others, and the ganglion itself is differently developed, but for what physiological purpose I know not. It is comparatively larger in the ox than in the horse, and sends more filaments to the iris. Four distinct filaments may be traced in the ox, but seldom more than two in the horse or the dog. To these filaments others of the ophthalmic, that have not passed through the ganglion, afterward join themselves; so that the ciliary are also minute compound nerves of motion and sensation.*

* "The best account, however, of this is given by Dr. Jonas Quain ('Quain's Anatomy,' p. 768). He considers the ganglion as a center of nervous influence—a little brain, as it were—and the filaments which some anatomists describe as composing, he speaks of as branches given out from it. 'It lies,' says he, 'within the orbit, about midway between the optic foramen and the globe of the eye, and is inclosed between the external rectus muscle and the optic nerve. It is exceedingly small and, owing to its being imbedded in the soft adipose tissue which fills the interstices of the different parts within the orbit, difficult to find. Its branches are the following: From its anterior border from sixteen to twenty filaments issue, which proceed forward to the surface of the sclerotic, and pierce it through minute foramina. These are the ciliary nerves. In their course to the globe of the eye they are joined by one or two filaments derived from the nasal nerve, but they do not form a plexus (an interlacement). They become, however, dispersed or divided into two fasciculi, one above and the other below the optic nerve, the latter being

"The ophthalmic nerve, after running between the rectus superior and the retractor muscles, gives a the more numerous. They pass between the choroid membrane and the contiguous surface of the sclerotic—lodged in grooves in the latter—and on reaching the ciliary ligament, pierce it, a few appearing to be lost in its substance, while all the rest pass inward and ramify in the iris. From the posterior border of the ganglion, which seems as if terminated by two angles, two branches issue, one of which passes backward and upward to the nasal branch of the ophthalmic nerve, appearing to be the medium of communication between the ganglion and the rest of the ganglial system, by being prolonged to the carotid plexus. The other, the shorter branch, passes downward and backward to the inferior oblique branch of the motor nerve of the eye.'

"For my own part," says Prof. Youatt, "I am now disposed to be very much of Dr. Quain's opinion. It was not fitting that the motions of the iris should be under the control of the will—they should respond to the varying intensity of the light."—*W. Youatt in "Veterinarian" for 1836, p. 49.*

Mons. Cuvier says: "It divides into two ramifications, one of which proceeds toward the optic, unites with the small branch of the third pair, and by this union produces a nervous enlargement called the lenticular or ophthalmic ganglion. This ganglion usually sends off the ciliary nerves, disposed in two bundles. They are each composed of several filaments, which enter the globe of the eye obliquely. The iris receives a great number of small ramifications from the ciliary nerves, which, after having perforated the sclerotic and passed around the choroides longitudinally, like ribbons, but without penetrating it, are lost."—*"Comparative Anatomy," Vol. II, p. 206.*

Prof. W. Percivall says: "Upon the outer side of the optic nerve, between it and that part of the motor oculi from which the branch nerves spring, is situated the ophthalmic ganglion. This little body is principally constituted of branches from the third pair, but it receives a filament or two from the sixth. The nervous threads transmitted by the ganglion surround the sheath of the optic nerve, and pursuing their course over it, penetrate the globe of the eye, and run to be dispersed upon the iris."—*"Anatomy of the Horse," p. 336.*

branch to the 'membrana nictitans,' and then takes a singular course. Some ramifications go to the frontal sinuses and the foramina, and, piercing the orbit of the eye for this purpose, present a beautiful view in young animals, particularly the sheep. The main branch then enters the cranium again through the internal orbital foramen, passes under the dura mater, returns through the cribriform plate, and ramifies on the membrane of the nose, sending some branches as low as the false nostril and alæ.

"The *superior maxillary nerve,* or second branch of the trigeminus, contains little that is peculiar to or has a practical tendency in quadrupeds. The different situation and conformation of the bones of the face cause the principal or only variation in the distribution of this branch in the biped and the quadruped. It leaves the cranium through the foramen rotundum, and at the base of the skull gives off small ramifications to the inner canthus of the eye, the antrum, and the two posterior grinder teeth. It also supplies the lateral portion of the nasal cavity through the sphenopalatine foramen, while filaments are given off from the origin of the trunk to the temporal muscle. A branch also runs along the upper border of the septum nasi to the palate, and a larger branch, which traverses the palate in company with its blood-vessels, passes through the foramen incisivum to the upper lip. The *main trunk* of the nerve now enters into the superior and exterior foramen, in the hiatus between the palatine bone and the tuberosity of the superior maxillary bone, leading into a bony canal (easily traced in the horse) between the maxillary sinus and the antrum, and appearing as a great pillar passing through the palatine sinuses in the ox. It traverses this canal, and at length emerges on the face through the foramen infra-orbitarium, and under the levator labii superioris muscle. It no sooner escapes from this canal than it forms the 'pes anserinus' (the goose's foot, for it divides something like the foot of this bird). It anastomoses with or receives numerous branches from the seventh pair, and forms an intricate plexus about the lower part of the face and muzzle. The nerves, however, are wisely and beautifully interwoven, for the lips, being the seat of touch, require all the flexibility and more than the sensibility of the human hand.

"The *inferior maxillary nerve*, or third branch of the trigeminus, emerges from the cranium through the foramen lacerum basis cranii, and very soon gives off *four* important branches. The first branch, reckoning posteriorly, proceeds backward below the condyle of the jaw, where it divides into two portions. The first runs up to the parotid gland, ramifies into many filaments, and unites with the seventh pair. It dips deep into and principally supplies the temporal muscle, and penetrates and is distributed through the masseter muscle. In this division there seems to be concentrated the greater part of the motor fibrils of the trigeminus, for these are muscles of extensive and powerful action. There are few muscles of the frame that are oftener or more powerfully employed than those concerned in mastication; but with the motor fibrils those of sensation are doubtless conjoined.

"The second branch is a long and slender one. It first dips into the pterygoideus muscle, which is supplied by it; consequently it is here also a motor as well as a sensitive nerve. It then passes around or behind the tuberosity of the upper jaw, supplying the buccinator muscle—possibly with sensitive fibrils alone, for others go to this muscle from the seventh pair. In the buccinator these fibrils are usually lost; but sometimes a few of them may be traced to the lower lip.

"The third branch, in the order of its being given off, is the *dental nerve*. This is generally considered the continuation of the trunk of the inferior maxillary nerve. It passes across the pterygoideus and enters a canal (the *dental canal*), on the inner face of the lower jawbone, near the upper edge, and at the bending or angle of the jaw. It takes its course along the interior of the bone (the canal), close to the roots of the teeth, and sends out filaments to each of them. Emerging through the lower maxillary foramen, it divides into two branches, one of which is distributed in numerous ramifications on the outside of the lower lip, and the other in fewer ramifications on the inside. These are evidently sensitive fibrils, the power of motion being derived from the seventh pair of nerves.

"The fourth branch in point of order, but which does not enter the 'dental canal,' is the *gustatory* or *lingual nerve*, the largest of the four. It is singularly flat, like a little ribbon. It runs along the inside of the lower jaw, and a branch of it enters a foramen in the jaw to supply the roots of the incisor teeth; but the main nerve, proceeding obliquely downward, gives fibrils to the submaxillary glands, and to the glands and muscles at the base of the mouth generally. These fibrils form true plexuses about the salivary glands and the muscles of the tongue. They anastomose freely with the twelfth pair (the linguales or motor nerve of the tongue), as the twelfth had already done with the seventh (the 'portio dura'). The gustatory branch penetrates the substance of the tongue between the stylo and genio-glossal muscles, passing obliquely to the surface of the tongue, and terminating in the papillæ. The papillæ, thus endowed with nervous influence, are the seat of the sense of taste."

Of the fifth nerve (in man and in the horse) Prof. Owen (quoting partly from Dr. Swan), says ("Odontography," vol. i, pp. lxv-vi):

"The nerves of the teeth are derived from the trigeminal, or fifth pair, of which the second division supplies those of the upper jaw, the third division those of the lower. In the human subject, the three dental branches of the infra-orbital nerve intercommunicate by their primary branches, from which, and from a rich plexus formed by secondary branches upon the membrane lining the antrum, two sets of nerves are sent off to the alveolar processes of the upper jaw; one set (*rami dentales*) supplies the teeth, the other (*rami gingivales*) the osseous tissue of the gums. The latter agree in number with the intervals of the teeth, as the proper dental nerves do with the teeth themselves. These two sets are not, however, so distinct but that some intercommunications are established between the fine branches sent off in their progress to the parts they are specially destined to supply. The *rami dentales* take the more direct course (through the middle part of the osseous tissue to the teeth) penetrate the orifices of the fangs, and form a rich plexus with rhomboidal meshes upon the coronal surface of the pulp, the peripheral elementary filaments returning into the plexus by loops. In the lower jaw the dental nerve, besides supplying the proper nerves to the teeth, also forms a rich plexus, in which it is joined by some branches from the division of the nerve that afterward escapes by the foramen mentale, and from this plexus the cancellous tissue of the bone and the vascular gums are supplied. \* \* \* \*

"In the horse the maxillary plexus is most developed above and between the alveoli of the three pre-molar teeth. It is less complex where it supplies the molar teeth, their alveoli, and the gums. In the lower jaw of the horse a very rich plexus begins to be formed in the cancellous substance of the bone by branches of the dental nerve, soon after its entry into the canal."

# VOCABULARY.

Note.—The definitions, where not otherwise credited, are from "Dunglison's Medical Dictionary."

## A.

Ala (plural, alæ). Projections from the median line; as the alæ nasi, alæ of the uterus, &c.

Albumen. An important organic compound. The characteristic ingredient in the white of egg; abounds in the serum of the blood, in chyle, lymph, skin, muscles, brain, and the juice of flesh; in small quantity in most vegetable juices, and in Bright's disease in considerable quantity in the urine. It is the foundation, says Liebig, of the whole series of peculiar tissues which constitute those organs which are the seat of all vital actions. *C. F. Chandler.*

Alve'olar Arches are formed by the margins or borders of the two jaws, which are hollowed by the alveoli.

Alveolar Artery, arises from the internal maxillary, descends behind the tuberosity of the upper jaw, and gives branches to the upper molar teeth, gums, periosteum, membrane of the maxillary sinus, and buccinator muscle.

Alveolar Border. The part of the jaws that is hollowed by the alveoli.

Alveolar Membranes are very fine membranes, situated between the teeth and alveoli, and formed by a portion of the sac which incloses the tooth before it pierces the gum. By some this membrane has been called the 'alveolo-dental periosteum.'

Alveolar Vein. This has a distribution similar to the artery.

ALVE′OLUS (pl. alveoli). The alveoli are the sockets of the teeth, into which they are, as it were, driven. Their size and shape are determined by the teeth which they receive, and they are pierced at the apex by small holes which give passage to the dental vessels and nerves.

ANASTOMO′SIS ('a mouth'). Communication between two vessels. By considering the nerves to be channels, in which a nervous fluid circulates, their communication likewise has been called anastomosis. By means of anastomoses, if the course of a fluid be arrested in one vessel, it can proceed along others.

ANISODAC′TYLE. Hoofed quadrupeds with toes (on the hind-feet at least) in uneven numbers, as one, three, or five, the latter being manifested by the Proboscidians. All these have a simple stomach and an enormous cæcum. Examples: Horse, tapir, rhinoceros, elephant. *R. Owen.*

ANTE′RIOR (*ante* 'before'). Great confusion has prevailed with anatomists in the use of the terms before, behind, &c.

(A practical definition of *anterior* appears to be (1) parts in *front*, supposing the body to be equally divided longitudinally from right to left; (2) parts nearest the operator, parts beyond being *posterior*.)

ANTRUM. A cavern. A name given to certain cavities in bones, the entrance to which is smaller than the bottom.

ANTRUM OF HIGHMORE. A deep cavity in the substance of the superior maxillary bone, communicating with the middle meatus of the nose. It is lined by a prolongation of the Schneiderian membrane.

ARACH′NOID MEMBRANE. A name given to several membranes, which, by their extreme thinness, resemble spider-webs. The moderns use it for one of the membranes of the brain, situate between the dura mater and pia mater. It is a serous membrane, composed of two layers, the external being confounded, in the greater part of its extent, with the dura mater, and, like it, lining the interior of the cranium and spinal canal; the other is extended over the brain, from which it is separated by the pia mater, without passing into the sinuosities between the convolutions, and penetrating into the interior of the brain by an opening at its posterior part, under the 'corpus callosum.' It forms a part of the investing

ARE'OLA. A diminutive of 'area.' Anatomists understand by areolæ the interstices between the fibers composing organs, or those existing between laminæ, or between vessels which interlace with each other.

ARGEN'TI NITRAS. Nitrate of silver; lunar caustic. The virtues of nitrate of silver are tonic and escharotic. It is given in chorea, epilepsy, &c.; locally, it is used in various cases as an escharotic. Dose, gr. 1-8 to gr. 1-4, in pill, three times a day.

ARMADIL'LO. (So called from being protected or *armed* by a scaly covering like the plate armor of the middle ages.) A genus of South American quadrupeds, belonging to the order of edentata, and characterized by a defensive armor of small bony plates, covering the head and trunk, and sometimes the tail. *Brande.*

ARTICULA'TION. The union of bones with each other, as well as the kind of union. Articulations are generally divided into two kinds—movable and immovable. The articulations are subject to a number of diseases, which are generally somewhat severe; they may be physical, as wounds, sprains, luxations, &c., or they may be organic, as ankylosis, extraneous bodies, caries, rheumatism, gout, &c.

AT'ROPHY. Progressive and morbid diminution in the bulk of the whole body or of a part. Atrophy is generally symptomatic. Any tissue or organ thus affected is said to be 'atrophied.'

AURIC'ULAR. (The ear.) That which belongs to the ear, especially the external ear.

## B.

BATRA'CHIA. An order of reptiles including toads, frogs, and salamanders. *Brande.*

One of the five great classes into which vertebrate animals are usually divided, though some writers have reduced the class to the rank of an order of reptiles, a class with which they are popularly confounded. The batrachians are cold-blooded and oviparous, and in most living species are without scales, and the blood is partly aërated through the skin. The young, for the most part, breathe by gills like those of fishes; they assume a fish-like form (as the tadpole), and finally, when adult, with few exceptions, lose their gills and breathe by lungs, like true or scaly reptiles. They generally have limbs, but not always. *Johnson's N. U. Cyc.*

BI'FURCATION. (A fork.) Division of a trunk into two branches, as the bifurcation of the trachea, aorta, &c.

BUCCAL. That which concerns the mouth, and especially the cheek.

## C.

CÆCUM. The blind gut; so called from its being perforated at one end only. That portion of the intestinal canal which is seated between the termination of the ileum and beginning of the colon, and which fills, almost wholly, the right iliac fossa, where the peritoneum retains it immovably. Its length is about three or four fingers' breadth. The ileo-cæcal valve, or valve of Bauhin, shuts off all communication between it and the ileum, and the 'Appendix vermiformis cæci' is attached to it.

In the horse the cæcum (water stomach) will hold four gallons. A horse will drink at one time a great deal more than his stomach will contain; but even if he drinks a less quantity, it remains, not in the stomach or small intestines, but passes to the cæcum, and is there retained, as in a reservoir, to supply the wants of the system. *Youatt.*

CAL'CULUS. A diminutive of 'caix,' a lime-stone. Calculi are concretions, which may form in every part of the animal body, but are most frequently found in the organs that act as reservoirs, and in the excretory canals. They are met with in the tonsils, joints, biliary ducts, digestive passages, lachrymal ducts, mammæ, pancreas, pineal gland, prostate, lungs, salivary, spermatic, and urinary passages, and in the uterus. The causes which give rise to them are obscure. Those that occur in reservoirs or ducts are supposed to be owing to the deposition of the substances, which compose them, from the fluid as it passes along the duct; those which occur in the substance of an organ are regarded as the product of some chronic irritation. Their general effect is to irritate, as extraneous bodies, the parts with which they are in contact, and to produce retention of the fluid whence they have been formed. The symptoms differ, according to the sensibility of the organ and the importance of the particular secretion whose discharge they impede. Their 'solution' is generally impracticable. Spontaneous expulsion or extraction is the only way of getting rid of them.

CANCEL'LI. 'Lattice-work.' The cellular or spongy texture of bone, consisting of numerous cells, communicating with each other. They contain a fatty matter, analogous to marrow. This texture is met with principally at the extremities of long bones, and some of the short bones consist almost wholly of it. It allows of the expansion of the extremities of bones, without adding to their weight, and deadens concussions.

CAN'ULA. Diminutive of canna, 'a reed.' A small tube of gold, silver, platinum, iron, lead, wood, elastic gum, or gutta-percha, used for various purposes in surgery.

CAP'ILLARY (from *capillus*, 'a hair'). Hair-like; small.

CAPILLARY VESSELS are the extreme radicles of the arteries and veins, which together constitute the capillary, intermediate, or peripheral vascular system—the methæ'mata blood channels of Dr. Marshall Hall (that is, the system of vessels in which the blood undergoes the change from venous to arterial, and conversely). They possess an action distinct from that of the heart.

CA'RIES. (Rottenness.) A disease of bones analogous to ulceration of soft tissues; a term for open ulcer of bone and chronic ostitis of its connective tissue, with solution of the earthy part. It begins as an inflammation, accompanied by periostitis, followed by exudation of new materials and softening. Sometimes the bone-cells are filled with a reddish fluid, and there are masses of tubercle. After caries has existed for some time the abscess bursts; aperture remains open, discharging a fluid and particles of bone; a probe is felt to sink into a soft, gritty substance—carious bone. Caries is molecular death of bone; necrosis is death of a mass of bone. *Willard Parker.*

CAROT'IDS. The great arteries of the neck, which carry blood to the head.

CAR'TILAGE. A solid part of the animal body, of a consistence between bone and ligament, which in the fetus is a substitute for bone, but in the adult exists only in the joints, at the extremities of the ribs, &c.

CER'VICAL. Everything which concerns the neck, especially the back part.

CHEVROTAIN'. A species of the genus Moschus, related to the deer, but having no horns, and otherwise peculiar. It is small, light, and graceful, and lives in the mountains of Asia, from the Altai to Java. *Dana.*

CHOROID MEMBRANE. A thin membrane, of a very dark color, which lines the sclerotic internally. It is situate between the sclerotic and retina, has an opening posteriorly for the passage of the optic nerve, and terminates anteriorly at the great circumference of the iris, where it is continuous with the ciliary processes. The internal surface is covered with a dark pigment, consisting of several layers of pigment cells. Its use seems to be to absorb the rays of light after they have traversed the retina.

CIL'IARY. Relating to the eyelashes, or to cilia. This epithet has also been applied to different parts, which enter into the structure of the eye, from the resemblance between some of them (the ciliary processes) and the eyelashes.

COLON. That portion of the large intestines which extends from the cæcum to the rectum. The colon is usually divided into four portions. 1. The right lumbar or ascending colon, situate in the right lumbar region, and beginning at the cæcum. 2. The transverse colon—transverse arch of the colon—the portion which crosses from the right to the left side, at the upper part of the abdomen. 3. The left lumbar or descending colon, extending from the left part of the transverse arch, opposite the outer portion of the left kidney, to the corresponding iliac fossa. 4. The iliac colon, or sigmoid flexure of the colon; the portion which makes a double curvature in the left iliac fossa, and ends in the rectum.

In the horse the colon is exceedingly large, and is capable of containing no less than twelve gallons of liquid or pulpy food. It is of considerable length; completely traversing the diameter of the abdominal cavity, it is then reflected upon itself, and retraverses the same space. *Youatt.*

COM'MISSURES. The point of union between two parts; thus the commissures of the eyelids, lips, &c., are the angles which they form at the place of union.

COMPARATIVE ANAT'OMY. The science which treats of the structure and relation of organs in the various branches of the animal kingdom, without a knowledge of which it is impossible to understand the beautifully progressive development of organization, necessary even for the full comprehension of the uses of many parts of the human body, which, apparently rudimentary and useless in man, are highly developed in other animals. This science is also the basis of physiology and the natural classification of animals.
*American Cyclopedia.*

CON'DYLE. An articular eminence, round in one direction, flat in the other. A kind of process, met with more particularly in the ginglymoid joints, such as the condyles of the occipital, inferior maxillary bone, &c.

CONGEN'ITAL (from *con* and *genitus*, 'begotten'). Diseases which infants have at birth; hence, congenital affections are those that depend on faulty conformation, as congenital hernia, congenital cataract, &c.

CONJUNCTI'VA MEMBRA'NA. A mucous membrane, so called because it unites the globe of the eye with the eyelids. It covers the anterior surface of the eye, the inner surface of the eyelids, and the 'caruncula lachrymalis.' It possesses great general sensibility, communicated to it by the fifth pair of nerves.

COPYRA'RA is the largest known quadruped of the order Rodentia, and belongs to the family Cavidæ. It is an aquatic animal, a native of South America, and feeds on vegetable food exclusively. Its dentition resembles that of the cavy, except that the grinding teeth are formed of many transverse plates, the number of plates increasing as the animal advances in age. It is inoffensive and easily tamed. The flesh is esteemed good food. It is somewhat smaller than the common hog. *Johnson's New Universal Cyclopedia.*

COR'PUSCLE. One of the ultimate morphological elements of the body. They exist at some time or other in all the tissues of the body, governing their vital actions. The white and red corpuscles of the blood, epithelial bodies and ganglionic nerve cells are examples. They are mainly composed of protoplasm and contain in their interior bodies called nuclei, in which are still smaller ones called nucleoli. *T. E. Satterthwaite.*

CORRELA'TION (mutual relation) OF FORCES (otherwise called 'Transmutation of Force or Energy'). A phrase of recent origin, employed to express the theory that any one of the various forms of physical force may be converted into one or more of the other forms. The cardinal point in this theory is the doctrine of heat and its relation to other agents, especially to mechanical motion. For example, the heat manifested when we rub two flat surfaces briskly against each other, is only our own muscular motion checked by the friction, and changed thereby into the heat which the surfaces reveal. On the other hand, this muscular motion is only the heat of our bodily frame expending itself in this way. In either case the energy has not been annihilated, but only transferred, and appears in a new form.

*Johnson's N. U. Cyc., article rerised by J. H. Seelye.*

CRURA. The plural of *crus*, 'a leg.' Applied to some parts of the body, from their resemblance to legs or roots, as the 'crura cerebri,' 'crura cerebelli,' &c.

CUL-DE-SAC. Any bag-shaped cavity, tubular vessel, or organ, open only at one end. *Dana.*

## D.

DENTAL CANAL. The bony canals through which the vessels and nerves pass to the interior of the teeth.

DENTAL CAVITY. A cavity in the interior of the teeth, in which is situate the dental pulp. (More properly the pulpal cavity.)

DENTAL PULP. The pultaceous substance, of a reddish-gray color, very soft and sensible, which fills the cavity of the teeth. It is well supplied with capillary vessels.

DENTIG'EROUS. Tooth-carrying, as dentigerous cysts; one containing teeth.

DERMAL. Relating or belonging to the skin.

DERMATOID or DERMOID. That which is similar to the skin. This name is given to different tissues which resemble the skin. The dura mater has been so called by some.

DETER'GENTS. Medicines which possess the power to deterge or cleanse parts, as wounds, ulcers, &c.

DIABE′TES. A disease characterized by great augmentation and often manifest alteration in the secretion of urine, with excessive thirst and progressive emaciation. The quantity of urine discharged in 24 hours is sometimes 30 pints and upward, each pint containing 2¼ ounces saccharine matter.

DI′APHRAGM. 1. A dividing membrane or thin partition, commonly with an opening through it. 2. The muscle separating the chest or thorax from the abdomen or lower belly; the midriff. *Webster.*

DIATH′ESIS. Disposition, constitution, affection of the body; predisposition to certain diseases rather than to others. The principal diatheses are the cancerous, scrofulous, scorbutic (pertaining to scurvy), rheumatic, gouty, and calculous.

DIVERTIC′ULUM. A blind tube branching out from the course of a larger one. An organ which is capable of receiving an unusual quantity of blood, when the circulation is obstructed or modified elsewhere, is said to act as a diverticulum.

In the marsupials only four teeth (one in each jaw on each side) are deciduous. The permanent set are developed from *diverticula* of the sacs which originated the first set. *Gill.*

DUGONG′. A herbivorous, cetaceous animal with a tapering body ending in a crescent-shaped fin. The fabled mermaid seems to have been founded on the dugong. *Gilbert. Brande.*

It is generally from 8 to 12 feet long, though it is said to sometimes attain the length of 25 feet. The upper lip is thick and fleshy and forms a kind of snout; the upper jaw bends downward almost to a right angle; eyes small, with a nictitating membrane; the skin is thick and smooth. Its flesh is said to resemble beef, and is prized as food. The oil is recommended as a substitute for cod-liver oil. *J.'s Cyc.*

DURA MATER. (Hard.) The outermost of three membranes enveloping the brain and spinal cord. Within the skull it so completely joins the bones that it may be regarded as their endosteum. Within the spinal canal it becomes a fibrous tube, separated from the vertebræ (which have no endosteum) by a loose, areolar, fatty tissue and a plexus of veins. It sends out sheaths for the nerves as they go through their foramina. It is usually studded, except in infancy, by minute whitish masses (Paccionian bodies) whose use is not known. Its inner surface is covered with pavement epithelium, and perhaps by the parietal layer of the arachnoid membrane. *Ibid.*

### E.

Econ'omy. By the term 'animal economy' is understood the aggregate of the laws which govern the organism. The word economy is also used for the aggregate of parts which constitute man or animals.

Edenta'ta. In natural history, an order of animals that are destitute of *front* teeth, as the armadillo and ant-eater. *Bell.*

Eden'tulus. One without teeth.

Em'bryo. The fecundated germ, in the early stages of its development in utero. At a certain period of its increase, the name 'fetus' is given to it, but at what period is not determined. Generally, the embryo state is considered to extend to the period of quickening.

Encephali'tis. This term has been used by some nosologists (classifiers of diseases) synonymously with 'cephalitis' and 'phrenitis.' By others it has been appropriated to inflammation of the brain, in contradistinction to that of the membranes.

E'ocene. In geology, a term applied to the earlier tertiary deposits, in which are a few organic remains of existing species of animals. Hence the term eocene (recent), which denotes the dawn of the existing state of things.

*Dana. Lyell. Mantell.*

In America the eocene strata contain numerous fossils, mostly marine mollusks, but also include some gigantic vertebrates, a carnivorous cetacean seventy feet in length, and a shark of which the teeth are sometimes six inches in length. The Wyoming beds have furnished the remains of a remarkable group of mammals, which are thought by Prof. Marsh to form a new order, and which he has named 'Dinocerata.' The largest of these (Dinoceras mirabilis) had the bulk of an elephant, and was provided with three pairs of horns and a pair of great saber-like canine teeth. *Johnson's N. U. Cyc.*

Epider'mis. A modification of the epithelium, molded to the papillary layer of the true skin; composed of agglutinated, flattened cells, which are developed in the liquor sanguinis, the latter being poured out on the true skin's external surface. In the deeper layers the cells are rounded or columnar, containing in most races of men more or less pigmentary matter, which gives the skin its various shades from black to white. It is penetrated by the ducts of the skin's sweat-glands and oil-glands; becomes hard in palms of hands; otherwise is soft. The hair and nails are modifications of it.

On leaves it is penetrated by the stomata, transmitting exhalations and absorbing carbonic acid, the most important part of plant food. *Ibid.*

EPITHE'LIUM. (Soft, delicate, tender.) The layer of cells lining serous (closed) and mucous (open) cavities, the mucous epithelium being continuous with the epidermis. (Mucous is formed by the bursting of epithelial cells.) *Ibid.*

ESOPH'AGUS. The gullet. Extends from pharynx to stomach.

ETHMOID. Sieve-like. The *ethmoid bone* is one of the eight bones which compose the cranium, so called because its upper plate is pierced by numerous holes. It is situate at the anterior, inferior, and middle part of the cranium.

EVOLU'TION. According to the hypothesis of evolution, in its simplest form, the universe as it now exists is the result of "an immense series of changes," related to and dependent upon each other, as successive steps, or rather growths, constituting a progress; analogous to the unfolding or evolving of the parts of a living organism. Evolution is defined by Herbert Spencer as consisting in a progress from the homogeneous to the heterogeneous, from general to special, from the simple to the complex; and this process is considered to be traceable in the formation of the worlds in space, in the multiplication of the types and species of plants and animals on the globe, in the origination and diversity of languages, literature, arts, and sciences, and in all the changes of human institutions and society. *Henry Hartshorne.*

The animal kingdom displays a unity of plan or a correlation of parts by which common principles are traced through the most disguising diversities of form, so that in aspect, structure, and functions the various tribes of animals pass into each other by slight and gradual transitions. The arm of a man, the fore limb of a quadruped, the wing of a bird, and the fin of a fish are homologous, that is, they contain the same essential parts, modified in correspondence with the different circumstances of the animal; and so with the other organs. Prof. Cope says: "Every individual of every species of a given branch of the animal kingdom is composed of elements common to all, and the differences which are so radical in the higher grades are but the modifications of the same elemental parts." *E. L. Youmans.*

EXFOLIA'TION (from *ex* and *folium*, 'a leaf'). By this is meant the separation of the dead portions of a bone, tendon, aponeurosis (a white shining membrane), or cartilage, under the form of lamellæ (small scales). Exfoliation is accomplished by the instinctive action of the parts, and its object is to detach the dead portions from those subjacent, which are still alive. For this purpose the latter throw out fleshy granulations, and a more or less abundant suppuration occurs, which tends to separate the exfoliated part—now become an extraneous body.

EXOSTO'SIS. An osseous tumor, which forms at the surface of bones, or in their cavities.

EXOSTOSIS DENTIUM. Exostosis of the teeth.

## F.

FERRU'GINOUS (chalyb'eate). Of or belonging to iron; containing iron. Any medicine into which iron enters, as chalybeate mixture, pills, waters, &c.

FE'TUS. See 'embryo.'

FIBER. An organic filament, of a solid consistence, and more or less extensible, which enters into the composition of every animal and vegetable texture.

FIL'AMENT. A thread. This word is used synonymously with fibril; thus we say a nervous or cellular filament or fibril.

FIS'TULA. 'A pipe or reed.' A solution of continuity (a division of parts previously continuous) of greater or less depth and sinuosity, the opening of which is narrow, and the disease kept up by an altered texture of parts, so that it is not disposed to heal. A fistula is 'incomplete' or 'blind' when it has but one opening, and 'complete' when there are two, the one communicating with an internal cavity, the other externally. It is lined in its whole course by a membrane which seems analogous to mucous membranes.

FOL'LICLE. A follicle or crypt is a small, roundish, hollow body, situate in the substance of the skin or mucous membranes, and constantly pouring the fluid which it secretes on their surfaces. The use of the secretion is to keep the parts on which it is poured supple and moist, and to preserve them from the action of irritating bodies with which they have to come in contact.

FORA'MEN. Any cavity pierced through and through. Also the orifice to a canal.

FOSSA. A cavity of greater or less depth, the entrance to which is always larger than the base.

FRÆNUM. A small bridle. A name given to several membranous folds, which bridle and retain certain organs.

FRONTAL BONE. A double bone in the fetus, single in the adult, situate at the base of the cranium, and at the superior part of the face.

FUNC'TION. The action of an organ or system of organs. Any act necessary for accomplishing a vital phenomenon. A function is a special office in the animal economy, which has as its instrument an organ or apparatus of organs.

FUNGUS. The mushroom order of plants. In pathology the word is commonly used synonymously with fungosity (mycosis).

FUNGUS HÆMATO'DES (Hæmatodes Fungus). An exceedingly alarming carcinomatous (cancerous) affection, which was first described with accuracy by Mr. John Burns, of Glasgow. It consists in the development of cancerous tumors, in which the inflammation is accompanied with violent heat and pain, and with fungus and bleeding excrescences.

## G.

GANG'LION. Nervous ganglions are enlargements or knots in the course of a nerve.

GASTRIC. Belonging or relating to the stomach.

GASTRIC JUICE. A fluid secreted from the mucous membrane of the stomach. It assists digestion.

GENTIAN WINE (vinum gentianæ compositum, or wine bitters). 'Gentiana Lutea' is the systematic name of the officinal gentian. The plant is common in the mountains of Europe. The root is almost inodorous, extremely bitter, and yields its virtues to ether, alcohol, and water. It is tonic and stomachic, and, in large doses, aperient. It is most frequently, however, used in infusion or tincture.

GEOL'OGY is that branch of natural science which treats of the structure of the crust of the earth and the mode of formation of its rocks, together with the history of physical changes and of life on our planet during the successive stages of its history. It has been *inferred* that its actual crust must be very thick, perhaps not less than 2,500 miles. Geology depends upon mineralogy for its knowledge of the constituents of rocks, and upon chemistry and physics for its knowledge of the laws of change; and in its study of fossil remains it is closely connected with the sciences of zoölogy and botany. A knowledge of geology lies at the base of physical geography, and is essential to the skillful prosecution of mining and other useful arts. *J. W. Dawson.*

The facts proved by geology are that during an immense but unknown period the surface of the earth has undergone successive changes; land has sunk beneath the ocean, while fresh land has risen up from it; mountain chains have been elevated; islands have been formed into continents, and continents submerged till they have become islands; and these changes have taken place, not once merely, but perhaps hundreds, perhaps thousands of times. *A. L. Wallace.*

Prof. Dana says the "earth was first a featureless globe of fire; then had its oceans and dry land; in course of time received mountains and rivers, and finally all those diversities of surface which now characterize it."

GLAND. (An acorn; a kernel.) Softish, granular, lobated organs, composed of vessels and a particular texture, which draw from the blood the molecules necessary for the formation of new fluids, conveying them externally by means of one or more excretory ducts. Each gland has an organization peculiar to it, but we know not the intimate nature of the glandular texture.

GUANA'CO. The 'Auchenia Huanaca,' a species of the genus of ruminant mammals to which the llama belongs. It inhabits the Andes, and is domesticated. It is allied to the camel.
*Webster.*

The guanaco is especially abundant in Patagonia and Chili, where it forms large flocks. It is about three feet high at the shoulders, and is extremely swift. In domestication it is ill-tempered, and has a disagreeable habit of ejecting saliva upon unwelcome visitors. In its wild state it seldom drinks water. Its flesh is edible and its skin valuable.

Johnson's N. U. Cyc.

## H.

HAVERSIAN CANALS. (Canals of Havers, nutritive canals, &c.) The canals through which the vessels pass to the bones. They are lined by a very fine lamina of compact texture, or are formed in the texture itself. There is generally one large nutritious canal in a long bone, situate toward its middle.

HIA'TUS. A foramen or aperture. Mouth. The vulva. Also yawning.

HISTOL'OGY is the branch of anatomy which treats of the minute structure of the *tissues* of which living beings are composed. It is divided into 'human histology,' which treats of the tissues of man; 'comparative histology,' which treats of the tissues of the lower animals, and 'vegetable histology,' which treats of the tissues of plants. Each of these divisions may be subdivided into 'normal' and 'pathological' histology, the first referring to the healthy tissues, the second investigating the changes they undergo in disease. *J. J. Woodward.*

HOOVE. A disease in cattle, consisting in the excessive inflation of the stomach by gas, ordinarily caused by eating too much green food. *Gardner.*

HYPER'TROPHY. The state of a part in which the nutrition is performed with greater activity, and which on that account at length acquires unusual bulk. The part thus affected is said to be hypertrophied or hypertrophous.

## I.

INFILTRA'TION. To filter; effusion. The accumulation of a fluid in the areolæ of a texture, and particularly in the areolar membrane. The fluid effused is ordinarily the 'liquor sanguinis,' sound or altered; sometimes blood or pus, fæces or urine. When infiltration of a serous fluid is general, it constitutes 'anasarca' (dropsy); when local, 'œdema.'

INTERSTI'TIAL. Applied to that which occurs in the interstices of an organ, as interstitial absorption, interstitial pregnancy, &c. (See 'Suppuration.')

INTRA-UTERINE. (*Intra*, 'within,' *uterus*, 'the womb.') That which takes place within the womb, as intra-uterine life.

Iris. So called from its resembling the rainbow in a variety of colors. A membrane, stretched vertically at the anterior part of the eye, in the midst of the aqueous humor, in which it forms a kind of circular, flat partition, separating the anterior from the posterior chamber. It is perforated by a circular opening called the pupil, which is constantly varying its dimensions, owing to the contractions of the fibers of the iris.

Isodac'tyle. Hoofed quadrupeds with toes in even number, as two or four, and which have a more or less complicated stomach, with a moderate-sized, simple cæcum. Examples: Ox, hog, peccary, hippopotamus. *R. Owen.*

## L.

Lach'rymal. Belonging to the tears. This epithet is given to various parts.

Lacunæ of Bone. Certain dark, stellate spots, with thread-like lines radiating from them, seen under a high magnifying power. These were first believed to be solid osseous corpuscles or cells (corpuscles of Purkinjé), but are now regarded as excavations in the bone, with minute tubes or canalic'uli proceeding from them and communicating with the Haversian canals. The lacunæ and canaliculi are fibers concentrated in the transit of nutrient fluid through the osseous tissue.

Lam'ina. A thin, flat part of a bone; a plate or table, as the cribriform lamina or plate of the ethmoid bone. Lamina and lamella are generally used synonymously, although the latter is properly a diminutive of the former.

Lesion. Derangement, disorder; any morbid change, either in the exercise of functions or in the texture of organs. 'Organic lesion' is synonymous with organic disease.

Lipo'ma. A fatty tumor of an encysted or other character.

Lipom'atous. Having the nature of lipoma, as a lipomatous mass.

Liquor Sang'uinis. A term given by Dr. B. Babington to one of the constituents of the blood, the other being the red particles. It is the effused material (called plasma, coagulable or plastic lymph, intercellular fluid, &c.), from which the cells obtain the constituents of the different tissues and secretions.

## M.

MALAR. Belonging to the cheek, as the malar bone.

MALAR PROCESS. Zygomatic process. (Cheek bone process.)

MASSETER. A muscle situate at the posterior part of the cheek, and lying upon the ramus of the lower jawbone. Its office is to raise the lower jaw and to act in mastication.

MAS'TODON. An extinct genus of quadrupeds. When alive it must have been twelve or thirteen feet high, and, including the tusks, about twenty-five feet long. The tusks measure ten feet eleven inches, about two and a half feet being implanted in the socket. According to Owen, the teeth are seven on each side, above and below. The molars have wedge-shaped, transverse ridges, the summits of which are divided by a depression lengthwise with the tooth, and subdivided into cones, more or less resembling the teats of a cow. In some species there are from three to five ridges to each posterior molar; in other species five or more. *O. C. Marsh.*

(The mastodon takes its name from the mastoid or nipple-like processes of its teeth.)

MASTOID. Having the form of a nipple.

MAX'ILLARY. Relating or belonging to the jaws.

MEA'TUS. A passage or canal.

MEDIAN LINE. A vertical line, supposed to divide a body longitudinally into two equal parts, the one right, the other left.

MED'ULLARY. Relating to the marrow, or analogous to marrow.

MEGATHE'RIUM. An extinct genus of Quaternary mammals. 'Megatherium Cuvieri,' from South America, exceeded the rhinoceros in size, its skeleton measuring eighteen feet in length. The vertebræ of the tail are very large and powerful, and that organ, with the hind-legs, seems to have formed a support for the heavy body, while the huge fore-legs were employed in breaking the branches from trees or tearing them down for food. There are four toes in front and two behind. The teeth, five above and four below on each side, resemble those of the sloths. They grew from persistent pulps, and are deeply implanted in the jaws; they have a grinding surface of triangular ridges, and were fitted for masticating coarse vegetable food. *O. C. Marsh.*

MEMBRANE. A name given to different thin organs, representing a species of supple and more or less elastic webs, varying in their structure and vital properties, and intended, in general, to absorb or secrete certain fluids, and to separate, envelop, and form other organs. Bichat has divided the membranes into simple and compound.

MEMBRA'NA NIC'TITANS. The 'haw' of the horse's eye. It is a triangular-shaped cartilage, concealed within the inner corner of the eye, and is black or pied. It is used by the horse, in lieu of hands, to wipe away dust, insects, &c. The eye of the horse has strong muscles attached to it, and one, peculiar to quadrupeds, by the aid of which the eye may be drawn back out of the reach of danger. When this muscle acts, the haw, which is guided by the eyelids, shoots across the eye with the rapidity of lightning, and thus carries off the offending matter. Its return is equally rapid. *Youatt.*

(Prof. Youatt denounces the practice of cutting out the haw as barbarous, that is, in ordinary cases of inflammation. He says that if farriers and grooms were compelled to walk for miles in the dust without being permitted to wipe or cleanse their eyes, they would feel the torture to which they often subject the horse.)

MI'OCENE. Literally, less recent. In geology, a term applied to the middle division of the tertiary strata, containing fewer shells of recent species than the Pliocene, but more than the Eocene. *Lyell.*

The Miocene is apparently the culminating age of the mammalia, so far as physical development is concerned, which accords with its remarkably genial climate and exuberant vegetation. In Europe the beds of this age present for the first time examples of the monkeys. Among carnivorous animals, we have cat-like creatures, one of which is distinguished from all modern animals of its group by the long, saber-shaped canines of its upper jaw, fitting it to pull down and destroy those large pachyderms which could have easily shaken off a lion or a tiger. Here also we have the elephants, the mastodon, a great, coarsely-built, hog-like elephant, some species of which had tusks both in the upper and lower jaw; the rhinoceros, the hippopotamus, and the horse, all of extinct species. *J. W. Dawson.*

MORPHOLOG'ICAL. That which has relation to the anatomical

conformation of parts. Applied at times to the alterations in the 'form' of the several parts of the embryo, in contradistinction to 'histological,' which is applied to the transformation by which the tissues are gradually generated. In comparative anatomy it is applied to the history of the modifications of forms which the same organ undergoes in different animals.

MORPHOL'OGY is that branch of zoölogy, in its widest sense, which treats of the general form (not outline) and organization of animals, and the principles involved, as well as the correspondence in the various forms of the several members and parts, so far as they are comparable in any structural characters, but entirely independent of the uses of the parts and organs. It thus contrasts with animal physiology, which treats of the organization in whole, so far as respects adaptation to surroundings, as well as the various parts and organs, so far as their uses and functions are concerned. To discover the utility of organization in diverse animal forms and the essential similarity in their mode of evolution, are the principal problems within the province of morphology. *Gill.*

MUCOUS MEMBRANE (lining of alimentary, respiratory, and genito-urinary tracts) consists of mucous membrane proper and submucous tissues. The first consists of secretory tubercles, follicles, and glands; the second of elastic connective tissue (capillary blood-vessels and nerve-filaments) by which the secretory surface is nourished. Its free surface is lined with epithelial cells, related to the mucous tissues beneath as the epidermic cells are to the skin; affords an extensive surface for the great functional glandular processes of nutritive absorption and the elimination of effete excretory products. Its special function is to secrete *mucus*, and thus protect its passages from the contact, attrition, and irritation of their moving contents. Mucus consists of water, mucosine, and salts. When rich in mucosine, it is viscid and tenacious; when salines predominate, it is scarcely more than transuded blood-serum. *E. D. Hudson, Jr.*

MUSK-DEER. A small deer of Central Asia; a timid creature of nocturnal habits, and is much hunted for its yield of musk, which is obtained from a sac beneath the abdomen, on the male alone. The flesh is esteemed, though that of the male is very rank and somewhat musky. It ranges from Siberia to Tonquin. *Johnson's N. U. Cyc.*

MUNTJAC, of India, Java, &c., a small deer, but little over two feet high. The males have small horns; the females are hornless. Their flesh is excellent. The Chinese muntjac, like the preceding, is often half domesticated, and is sometimes bred in European parks. *Johnson's N. U. Cyc.*

MYL'ODON. An extinct edentate animal, allied to the megatherium. *Lyell.*

## N.

NAR'WHAL, or SEA-UNICORN. It is most nearly related to the white whale. Belonging to an order in which many of the members never develop teeth at all, it, of all animals, is supplied with a tooth altogether out of proportion to its size, and it is, moreover, developed in utter contravention of the rules of bilateral symmetry, which in every known case among vertebrates govern the production of the teeth. In both sexes the lower jaw is edentulous. The male, however, is provided, on the left side of the upper jaw, with a tusk from eight to ten feet long. It is straight, spirally grooved externally, and hollowed within into a persistent pulp-cavity. On the right side the corresponding tooth generally remains hidden, smooth, and solid, within the jaw. In addition to these, there are two small rudimentary molars concealed in the upper jaw. The narwhal, which is considered one of the greatest curiosities of natural history, attains to a length of fifteen feet. Its single spiracle or blow-hole is situated on the top of the head. *E. C. H. Day.*

NECRO'SIS, or death of a bone, corresponds to mortification of the soft structures, and is as distinct from caries as mortification is from ulceration. Necrosis is divided into four varieties, namely: 1. The scrofulous. 2. The superficial, or that which involves the outer lamellæ, and presents itself in the flat and long bones. 3. That form which destroys the internal part of a bone, and in which the outer shell is not affected. 4. That in which the whole thickness of the bone dies. *W. Williams.*

## O.

ODONTAL'GIA. Toothache.

ODONTOG'ENY. Generation or mode of development of the teeth.

**ODONTOG′RAPHY.** A description of the teeth.

**ODON′TOID.** Tooth-shaped.

**ODONTOL′ITHOS.** A sort of incrustation, of a yellowish color, which forms at the coronæ of the teeth, and is called 'tartar.' It consists of 79 parts of phosphate of lime, $12\frac{1}{2}$ of mucus, 1 of a particular salivary matter, and $7\frac{1}{2}$ of animal substance, soluble in chlorohydric acid. A species of infusoria, 'denticola hominis,' has been found in it.

**ODONTOL′OGY.** An anatomical treatise of the teeth.

**ORAL.** Relating to the mouth or to speech.

**ORAL EPITHE′LIUM.** See 'Epithelium.'

**ORNITHORHYN′CHUS.** An effodient (digging), monotrematous mammal, with a horny beak resembling that of a duck, and two merely fibrous cheek teeth on each side of both jaws, not fixed in any bone, but only in the gum; with pentadactylous (five-fingered) paws, webbed like the feet of a bird, and formed for swimming, and with a spur in the hinder feet, emitting a poisonous liquid from a reservoir in the sole of the foot, supplied by a gland situated above the pelvis, and by the side of the spine. The animal is covered with a brown fur. It is found only in New Holland, and is sometimes called Water Mole. *Bell.*

As the name of the order imports, the alimentary, urinary, and reproductive organs open into a common cloaca, as in birds; mammary glands are present, secreting milk for the young, which are born blind and naked; there are no prominent nipples, and the mammary openings are contained in slits in the integument; M. Verreaux says the young, when they are able to swim, suck in the milk from the surface of the water, into which it is emitted. *American Cyc.*

'Duck-Bill,' the English name of the Ornithorhynchus paradoxus, found in Van Diemen's land and Australia. In its bill-like jaws, its spurs, its monotrematous character, its non-placental development, and its anatomy, it appears to be a connecting link between birds and mammals. The Duck-Bill is the only animal of its genus. It is about fifteen inches long; it climbs trees with facility, and digs burrows, often thirty feet long, in the river bank, with one opening above and another below water. It inhabits ponds and quiet streams, swimming about with its head somewhat elevated, often diving for its food, which consists of insects and other small aquatic animals. *Johnson's N. U. Cyc.*

Of all the mammalia yet known, the Ornithorhynchus seems the most extraordinary in its conformation, exhibiting the perfect resemblance of the beak of a duck engrafted on the head of a quadruped. *Dr. Shaw.*

According to Ernst H. Haeckel, these animals "are becoming less numerous year by year, and will soon be classed, with all their blood relations, among the extinct animals of our globe."

Os. A bone; also a mouth.

Osteol'ogy. The part of anatomy which treats of bones.

Osteo-sarco'ma. Disease of the bony tissue, which consists in softening of its laminæ, and their transformation into a fleshy substance, analogous to that of cancer, accompanied with general symptoms of cancerous affection. The word has also often been used synonymously with 'spina ventosa.'

O'varies (*ovum*, egg). The two organs in oviparous animals in which the ova, the generative product of the female, are formed. They are termed by Galen 'testes muliebres,' since they are in women the analogues of the testes in men. The ovaries in adult women are situated on either side of the uterus, in the iliac fossæ; they are included in the two pelvic duplicatures of the peritoneum, which are called the broad ligaments. Each ovary is also attached by a round, fibrous cord—the ovarian ligament—to the side of the uterus, and by a lesser fibrous cord to the fringed edge of the Fallopian oviduct. The ovary is an oblong, ovoid, flattened body, of a whitish color and uneven surface. It is $\frac{1}{8}$ to $\frac{1}{2}$ an inch thick, $\frac{3}{4}$ of an inch wide, and 1 inch to $1\frac{1}{2}$ long; it weighs from 1 to 2 drachms. *E. Darwin Hudson, Jr.*

Oze'na. An affection of the pituitary membrane, which gives occasion to a disagreeable odor similar to a crushed bed-bug.

## P.

Paleontol'ogy. The study of ancient beings. The science which treats of the evidences of organic life upon the earth during the different past geological periods of its history. These evidences consist in the remains of plants and animals imbedded or otherwise preserved in the rocky strata or upon their surfaces, and in other indications of animal existence, such as trails, footprints, burrows, and coprolitic or other organic material found in the rocks. Pythagoras, Plato, Aristotle, and other ancients, allude to the existence of marine shells at a distance from the sea: it was considered conclusive evidence that the rocks containing them had formerly been submerged beneath the ocean. *Am. Cyc.*

PAPIL′LA. The end of the nipple, or an eminence similar to a nipple.

The minute elevations of the surface of the skin, tongue, &c. They serve to increase the extent of surface for vascular distribution, or subserve sensitive or mechanical purposes. Some contain one or more vascular loops; others, nervous elements. Some are surmounted by dense epithelial filaments, as those which give the roughness to the tongue.

*Webster.*

PAR′ASITE. Parasites are plants which attach themselves to other plants, and animals which live in or on the bodies of other animals, so as to subsist at their expense. The mistletoe is a parasitic plant, the louse a parasitic animal.

PARI′ETES. A name given to parts which form the inclosure or limits of different cavities of the body, as the parietes of the cranium, chest, &c.

PAROT′ID. ('About the ear.') The largest of the salivary glands, seated under the ear and near the angle of the lower jaw. It secretes saliva.

PATHOL′OGY. The branch of medicine whose object is the knowledge of disease. It has been defined 'diseased physiology,' and 'physiology of disease.' It is divided into general and special. The first considers diseases in common; the second the particular history of each. It is subdivided into internal and external, or medical and surgical.

PELVIS The part of the trunk which bounds the abdomen below.

PERIODONTI′TIS. Inflammation of the membrane that lines the socket of a tooth.

PERIOS′TEUM. The periosteum is a fibrous, white, resisting medium, which surrounds the bones everywhere, except the teeth at their coronæ (crowns), and the parts of other bones that are covered with cartilage. The external surface is united, in a more or less intimate manner, to the adjoining parts by areolar tissue. Its inner surface covers the bones, whose depressions it accurately follows. It is united to the bone by small fibrous prolongations, and especially by a prodigious quantity of vessels, which penetrate their substance. It unites the bones to the neighboring parts, and assists in their growth, either by furnishing, at its inner surface, an albuminous exudation, which becomes cartilaginous and at length ossifies, or by supporting the vessels which penetrate them to carry the materials of their nutrition.

PETROUS. Resembling stone; having the hardness of stone.

PHLEGMON. Inflammation of the areolar texture, accompanied with redness, circumscribed swelling, increased heat and pain, which, at first, is tensive and lancinating and afterward pulsatory and heavy. It is apt to terminate in suppuration.

PIA MATER (tender mother), so named because it nourishes the nerve-centers. The innermost covering of the brain and spinal cord; a fine plexus of blood-vessels, dipping into the brain's convolutions, forming the velum interpositum in the third and the choroid plexus in the fourth ventricle. A small part (over the crura and pons) is not very vascular, but tough and fibrous, while that of the spinal cord, with which it is intimately connected and of which it is the neurilemma, is still less vascular. It is partly composed of longitudinal fibrous bundles, and is abundantly supplied with nerves and lymphatics. The tunica vasculosa of the testes is also called pia mater. *Johnson's N. U. Cyc.*

PITU'ITARY. Concerned in the secretion of muscus or phlegm.

PITUITARY MEMBRANE. The mucous membrane which lines the nasal fossæ, and extends to the cavities communicating with the nose. It is the seat of smell.

PLAS'MA. See 'Liquor Sanguinis.'

PLEISTOCENE. A term used to denote the newest tertiary deposits. *Johnson's N. U. Cyc.*

PLI'OCENE. In geology, the term applied to the most modern of tertiary deposits, in which most of the fossil shells are of recent species. *Lyell.*

With regard to animal life, the Pliocene continues the conditions of the Miocene, but with signs of decadence. The Pliocene was terminated by the cold or Glacial period, in which a remarkable lowering of temperature occurred over all the northern hemisphere, accompanied, at least in a portion of the time, by a very general and great subsidence, which laid all the lower part of our continent under water. This terminated much of the life of the Pliocene, and replaced it with boreal and arctic forms, some of them, like the great hairy Siberian mammoth and the woolly rhinoceros, fit successors of the gigantic Miocene fauna. *J. W. Dawson.*

POL'YPUS. A name given to tumors which occur in mucous membranes especially, and which have been compared to certain zoöphytes. Polypi may form on every mucous membrane. They vary much in size, number, mode of adhesion, and intimate nature. Fibrous polypi are of a dense, compact texture and whitish color. They contain few vessels and do not degenerate into cancer. The scirrhous or carcinomatous are true cancerous tumors, painful and bleeding.

PONS VAROLII. An eminence at the upper part of the medulla oblongata, first described by Varolius. It is formed by the union of the crura cerebri and crura cerebelli.

POSTE'RIOR. Opposed to 'anterior,' which see.

PTER'YGOID. A name given to two processes at the inferior surface of the sphenoid bone, the two laminæ which form them having been compared to wings.

PYLOR'IC. That which relates to the 'pylorus.' An epithet given to different parts.

PYLO'RUS. A 'gate,' a 'guardian.' The lower or right orifice of the stomach is called 'pylorus' because it closes the entrance into the intestinal canal, and is furnished with a circular, flattened, fibro-mucous ring, which causes the total closure of the stomach during digestion in that organ. It is a fold of the mucous and muscular membranes of the stomach, and is the 'pyloric muscle' of some authors.

## Q.

QUADRUMA'NA. (*Quatuor,* 'four,' and *manus,* 'hand.') A name employed by Blumenbach (in 1791) as an ordinal designation for the monkeys, lemurs, and related types, man having been isolated as the representative of a peculiar order named Bimanus. The views thus expressed were for a long time predominant; but a closer study of the structure of the forms indicated by those names has convinced almost all living naturalists that they were erroneously separated, and the two types are now generally combined in one order named Primates, under which head man and the monkeys are combined together in one sub-order (Anthropoidea), and contrasted with the lemurs, which constitute another sub-order (Prosimiæ). *Theodore Gill.*

## R.

RECTUM. The third and last portion of the great intestine. It forms the continuation of the sigmoid flexure of the colon, occupies the posterior part of the pelvis, and extends from the sacro-vertebral articulation to the coccyx (rump or crupper bone), before which it opens outward by the orifice called the 'anus.'

RÉG'IME. Mode of living; government, administration.

REG'IMEN. The rational and methodical use of food and of everything essential to life, both in a state of health and disease. It is often restricted in its meaning to 'diet.' It is sometimes used synonymously with hygiene (health).

RU'MINANT. A division of animals having four stomachs, the first so situated as to receive a large quantity of vegetable matter coarsely bruised by a first mastication, which passes into the second, where it is moistened and formed into little pellets; these the animal has the power of bringing again to the mouth, to be rechewed, after which it is swallowed into the third stomach, from which it passes into the fourth, where it is finally digested. *Webster.*

(Several well authenticated cases of human beings who *ruminated* their food are on record.)

## S.

SARCO'MA. Any species of excrescence having a fleshy consistence.

SCHNEIDERIAN MEMBRANE. See 'Pituitary membrane.'

SCLEROT'IC. A heavy, resisting, opaque membrane, of a pearly white color and fibrous nature, which covers nearly the posterior four-fifths of the globe of the eye, and has the form of a sphere truncated before.

SELLA TUR'CICA. (Turkish saddle.) A depression at the upper surface of the sphenoid bone, which is bounded, anteriorly and posteriorly, by the clinoid processes, and lodges the pituitary gland. It is so called from its resemblance to a Turkish saddle.

SEPTUM. A part intended to separate two cavities from each other, or to divide a principal cavity into several secondary cavities.

SEROUS. Thin, watery. Relating to the most watery portion of animal fluids, or to membranes that secrete them.

SOL'IPED. An animal whose hoof is not cloven; one of a group of animals with undivided hoofs; a solidungulate. *Webster.*

The family 'Solipeda' consists of several species of horse, namely, the ass, the mule, and the quagga. *Youatt.*

SPHENOID. Wedge-shaped.

SPHENOID BONE. An azygous (single) bone, situate on the median line, at the base of the cranium. It articulates with all the bones of that cavity, supporting them and strengthening their union. Its form is singular, resembling a bat with its wings extended.

SPINA VENTO'SA. See 'Osteo-sarcoma.'

STYLOID. (A style, a peg, a pin.) Shaped like a peg or pin.

SUBMAX'ILLARY (from *sub*, 'under,' *maxilla*, 'the jaw'). That which is seated beneath the jaw.

SUPPURA'TION. Formation or secretion of pus. It is a frequent termination of inflammation, and may occur in almost any of the tissues. This termination is announced by slight chills, by remission of the pain, which, from being lancinating, becomes heavy; by a sense of weight in the part, and, when the collection of pus can be easily felt, by fluctuation. When pus is thus formed in the areolar membrane, and is collected in one or more cavities, it constitutes an 'abscess.' If it be formed from a surface exposed to the air, it is an 'ulcer,' and such ulcers we are in the habit of establishing artificially in certain cases of disease.

SUPRA. A common Latin prefix, signifying 'above.'

SUTURE. A kind of immovable articulation, in which the bones unite by means of serrated edges, which are, as it were, dovetailed into each other. The articulations of the greater part of the bones of the skull are of this kind.

SYM'PHYSIS. A union of bones. The bond of such union. The aggregate of means used for retaining bones *in situ* (natural situations) in the articulations. The name symphysis has, however, been more particularly appropriated to certain articulations, as the 'symphysis pubis,' 'sacro-iliac symphysis,' &c.

## T.

**Teleosts** (or **Teleostei**). The name of that sub-class of fishes which embraces the great majority of living species, and so designated (by Johannes Müller) on account of the ossified condition of the skeleton in all the representatives of the group. *Theodore Gill.*

**Teratol'ogy.** A treatise on monsters.

**Ter'tiary.** Third; of the third formation. In geology, a series of strata, more recent than the chalk, consisting of sandstones, clay beds, limestones, and frequently containing numerous fossils, a few of which are identical with existing species. It has been divided into Eocene, Miocene, and Pliocene, which see. *Dana.*

**Tinctu'ra Myrrhæ.** (Tincture of Myrrh.) Tonic, deobstruent (removing obstructions), antiseptic (opposed to putrefaction), and detergent. It is chiefly used in gargles, and is applied to foul ulcers, spongy gums, &c.

**Tissue.** By this term, in anatomy, is meant the various parts which, by their union, form the organs, and are, as it were, their anatomical elements. 'Histological anatomy' is the anatomy of the tissues, which are the seat of the investigations of the pathological anatomist. The best division, indeed, of diseases would be according to the tissues mainly implicated.

**Tox'odon.** A gigantic, pachydermatous quadruped, now extinct, having teeth bent like a bow. *Brande.*

**Transuda'tion.** (To sweat.) The passage of a fluid through the tissue of any organ, which may collect in small drops on the opposite surface, or evaporate from it.

**Trephine'.** The instrument which has replaced the trepan in some countries. It consists of a simple, cylindrical saw, with a handle placed transversely, like that of a gimlet; from the center of the circle described by the saw a sharp little perforator, called the center-pin, projects. The center-pin is capable of being removed, at the surgeon's option, by means of a key. It is used to fix the instrument until the teeth of the saw have made a groove sufficiently deep for it to work steadily.' The pin must then be removed. Sometimes the pin is made to slide up and down, and to be fixed in any position, by means of a screw.

TRO'CAR. An instrument used for evacuating fluids from cavities, particularly in ascites (serous fluid in the abdomen, or, more properly, dropsy of the peritoneum), hydrocele (watery tumors), &c. A trocar consists of a perforator, or stylet, and a canula. The canula is so adapted to the perforator that, when the puncture is made, both enter the wound with facility; the perforator being then withdrawn, the fluid escapes through the canula.

TUBERCLE. *Miliary tubercles* are minute, bright, rounded, translucent particles, called granula, granulations, &c. When they coalesce, forming larger bodies and undergo a change of color they are known as *crude* or *yellow* tubercles. As age advances, the center is apt to be occupied by a giant cell, a large multi-nucleated body, whose boundaries and processes are hard to define, because they shade off gradually into the surrounding tissue. They are the result of an inflammatory process, because they can be produced by the introduction of mechanical irritants. In some instances we have reason to believe miliary tubercles may become organized and a cure result. Tuberculosis is hereditary, and there is some good evidence to prove it is contagious; it is also inoculable, and "breeds true," always producing its kind, if it produces anything, but it has not been satisfactorily proved to have a specific virus. *T. E. Satterthwaite.*

(Dr. Koch of Berlin says (1882) tuberculosis is caused by minute, rod-shaped parasites (bacilli); that he has inoculated animals with them, producing tuberculosis; that he has dried the sputum of phthisical patients for two months and has bred the parasites artificially for several generations without their losing the power of inoculation; that when the sputum is dried the air is infected; that bovine and human tuberculosis are identical; that tuberculosis can be given to man by the milk (perhaps flesh also) of tuberculous cows. The parasites are about $\frac{1}{6000}$th of an inch in length.)

TUNIC. An envelop; as the tunic of the eye, stomach, bladder.

TURGES'CENCE. Superabundance of humors in a part. 'Turgescence of bile' was formerly used to denote the passage of that fluid into the stomach and its discharge by vomiting.

TYMPANI'TES. A flatulent distention of the belly; tympany. Also inflammation of the lining membrane of the middle ear.

## U.

UN'GULATE. Shaped like a hoof. Having hoofs, as ungulate quadrupeds. *Webster.*

U'VEA (from *uvea*, a grape). The choroid coat of the eye; the posterior layer of the iris.

U'VEOUS. Resembling a grape; applied to the choroid coat of the eye.

## V.

VAS'CULAR. That which belongs or relates to vessels—arterial, venous, lymphatic—but generally restricted to blood-vessels only. Full of vessels.

VELUM PALA'TI. The soft palate.

VER'TEBRÆ. The bones which form the spinal column.

VIS'CUS (plural, vis'cera). One of the organs contained in the great cavities of the body; any one of the contents of the cranium, thorax, or abdomen; in the plural, especially applied to the contents of the abdomen, as the stomach, intestines, &c. *Webster.*

VIT'REOUS. Of, pertaining to, or derived from glass. The vitreous humor of the eye is so called because it resembles melted glass.

## Z.

ZOÖL'OGY. That part of biology (science of life) which relates to animal life, and, as generally understood, the science which treats of the structure, classification, distribution, habits, and derivation of living animals. In its broadest sense, however, zoölogy includes the structure, relations, and histories of extinct as well as living forms; but this branch of the science is generally considered by itself under the title of 'paleontology.' The derivation and life-histories of many groups of animals have been found written in the records of the past, and many mysteries, not only of relation but of structure, have been solved by going back to find dwarfed organs in full development and widely-separated forms linked together. The zoölogy of the future will therefore include the animal life of both the past and the present.

*J. S. Newberry.*

ZYGOMAT'IC. That which relates to the zygoma or cheek bone.

# APPENDIX.

## RECENT DISCOVERIES OF FOSSIL HORSES.

### BY J. L. WORTMAN.

THE contributions to the knowledge of the extinct Perissodactyla,* made during the last two or three years in this country, are of an important character, since they demonstrate the actual existence of types heretofore hypothetically assumed. The living representatives, the horse, tapir, and rhinoceros, constitute but a small fraction of this large order when compared with the fossil forms already known. One of these, however, the horse, displays the most specialized structure to be found within the limits of the order.

Many years have elapsed since the first discovery in the Tertiary rocks of Europe of horse-like remains, which are regarded by paleontologists in the light of direct ancestry of existing equines. Since then the discovery of the remains of these animals in the same geological horizons in this country, by Drs. Hayden and Leidy, has strengthened the belief in the descent of the horse from very different ancestral types. Entire skeletons, obtained from the "bone beds" of the West, display

---

* Odd-toed. The Perissodactyla may be defined as mammals having both pair of limbs fully developed and adapted for walking or running, the toes having terminal phalanges, incased in strong corneous sheaths, developed as hoofs. These characters, however, apply to two other orders also, the Artiodactyla (cloven-hoofed or even toed), and the Amblypoda (short-footed), both of which, however, possess many anatomical differences from the Perissodactyla, particularly in the structure of their hind limbs.

their osteological characters to such an extent as to leave no doubt as to the correct determination of their true affinities.

It is much to be regretted, however, that many of these animals have received different names from different authors, a fact specially conducive to confusion in the nomenclature of the science. It appears that the only way to obviate this difficulty is by strict adherence to priority in the employment of a name, provided it is accompanied by a competent description, and the use of such characters as will distinguish the animal named from its nearest allies. If unaccompanied by these differential characters, it is a *nomen nudum*, and can have no claim whatever to rank with those that have been properly defined. I mention these facts with the hope of establishing a criterion by which to judge which name it is proper to retain and which it is proper to discard; and, to elucidate the subject, I will gives the names of a few animals that have been discovered during the past forty years.

In 1841 Prof. Richard Owen described the remains of a Lophiodon-like* animal, from the London clay of Eocene age, to which he gave the name *Hyracotherium*.[†] Subsequently he described a nearly allied genus, from the same deposit, under the name *Pliolophus*.[‡] In *Hyracotherium* the molar and premolar teeth are different, both above and below. In *Pliolophus* the last, or fourth inferior premolar, is like the first true molar, a character which separates the two genera satisfactorily. The specimens described by Prof. Owen do not display clearly the number of digits either possessed, but he expresses the opinion that *Pliolophus* has three toes on the posterior limbs.

---

\* The Lophiodons were first described by Cuvier. They were allied to the tapir. They derive their name from the structure of the true molars, which have their crowns crossed transversely by two crests or ridges of dentine, covered with a layer of enamel. The last lower molar has also a small posterior lobe. The premolars are more simple in structure and compressed, resembling the first premolars of the tapir. The upper molars also resemble those of the tapir, but approach in some respects those of the rhinoceros. The diastema, or toothless interval between the canine and premolar teeth, was much shorter than in the tapir. Several species have been described from the Eocene of France and England, but little is known of the skull or skeleton. No true Lophiodon is yet certainly known in this country.—*O. C. Marsh.*

† Transactions London Geological Society, 1841, pp. 203–208.

‡ Loc. Cit., pp. 54–72, 1858.

In 1872 Prof. O. C. Marsh found the remains of an animal in this country in deposits of Eocene age to which he applied the name *Orohippus*.\* This genus was originally founded on the molar teeth, which he compared with those of *Anchitherium*. He subsequently ascertained that it possessed four toes on the anterior and three on the posterior limbs.† He also *proposed* another genus under the name of *Eohippus*, ‡ which he compared with *Orohippus*, stating that the last inferior premolar is like the first true molar, a character which at once distinguishes it from *Hyracotherium*. As he assigns no other dental characters to this genus sufficient to separate it from *Pliolophus*, with which, according to his description, it otherwise agrees, and as the digital formula in the Lophiodons generally is 4—3, the two names must be regarded as synonymous. This may likewise be said of the genus *Orotherium*,§ which Prof. Marsh distinguishes by the bifid condition of the antero-internal lobe of the inferior molars. This character is also ascribed to a number of molar teeth discovered by Dr. Joseph Leidy in the Bridger Eocene, which he referred to the genus *Lophiotherium*, a near ally of *Pliolophus*. But as this is a character of very doubtful generic value in this group of animals, these names must be regarded as synonymous with *Pliolophus*.

Assuming then that the most generalized form in the ancestry of the horse hitherto known was Hyracotherium, with a digital formula of 4—3 and teeth of the Lophiodon pattern, we are now prepared to take a step backward to the primitive five-toed ancestor, *Phenacodus*. But before entering on a discussion of this interesting form, it is necessary to mention the discovery of another genus, from the Lower Eocene beds of Wyoming, which proves to be a near ally of *Hyracotherium*. This genus Prof. Cope calls *Systemodon*,‖ and assigns as his reasons for separating it from *Hyracotherium* the circumstance that it dis-

---

\* American Journal Science and Arts, 1872.

† Loc. Cit., p. 247, 1874.

‡ Loc. Cit., Nov., 1876. The genera Orohippus, Eohippus, Miohippus, and Pliohippus have not in my estimation been distinguished from genera previously described; hence my reasons for adopting names more in accordance with the prevailing nomenclature of the science.

§ Loc. Cit., 1872.

‖ American Naturalist, 1881, p. 1018.

plays no diastemata (spaces) behind the superior canines, while in the latter there are two. This fossil (from New Mexico) was first described by him under the name *Hyracotherium tapirinum*, but the discovery of better specimens demonstrates its claim to the rank of a new genus.

## PHENACODUS.

Phenacodus, one of the most important of recent paleontological discoveries, was first made known by Prof. Cope in 1873,* from several molar teeth which he obtained from the New Mexican Wasatch. Its systematic position in the mammalian class was, however, involved in considerable uncertainty till the discovery of the greater part of the skeletons of two distinct species of this genus by the writer in the Wyoming Wasatch during the summer of 1881, which afforded Prof. Cope the means of determining its true position and elucidating the many important and interesting points its osteology teaches.† It possesses five well developed toes in functional

---

* Paleontological Bulletin, No. 17, Oct. 1873, p. 3.

† Prior to the discovery of these skeletons no characters had been found among the Ungulata which indicate a group connecting the Perissodactyla with the elephants and hyrax.* But it is now necessary to create a new order, which Prof. Cope designates the *Condylarthra*. (Paleontological Bulletin, No. 34, Dec. 1881, p. 177). The characters on which this division reposes are found in the carpus and the astragalus (hock or ankle bone) and their manner of articulation. The *Perissodactyla* are distinguished by the fact that the scaphoid articulates with two bones below, and the astragalus articulates inferiorly by two nearly flat facets with the cuboid and navicular bones. They are divisible into ten families, including forty-eight genera, variously distributed throughout geologic time; but as only four of these families concern us for the present, I will spare the memory of the reader by not discussing the classification of the others. The first to which attention may be directed is the *Lophiodontidæ*, embracing eight well de-

---

* A gray-haired, rabbit-sized pachyderm, with 4 toes on the forefeet, 3 on the hind, a mere tubercle for a tail, molars resembling (in miniature) those of the rhinoceros, 2 large, triangular, curved, tusk-like incisors in the upper jaw, and 4 straight ones in the lower. Cuvier says the upper jaw, in youth, has 2 small canines, but Marsh's dental formula is: Incisors, 1—2, 1—2; canines, 0—0, 0—0; premolars, 4—4, 4—1; molars, 3—3, 3—3 -31. There are several species, the African being able to climb a tree. The Cape hyrax is called the *rock-badger* or *rock-rabbit*. The hyrax was long classed among the rodents, and was also called a miniature rhinoceros. There are various affinities between the elephant and some rodents—(1) in the size of the tusks; (2) in the molars being often formed of parallel laminæ; (3) in the form of several of their bones.

use on all the feet, of which the first is the smallest; the median is the largest and is symmetrical within itself. The feet are considerably shortened and were probably semiplantigrade; in fact the feet of this animal constitute an approach to the Amblypoda.* The dental formula is: Incisors, 3—3,

---

fined genera, which are not positively known to have existed later than the upper Eocene epoch. It may be recognized (1) by the possession of four toes on the anterior and three on the posterior limbs; (2) by the molar and premolar teeth being different; (3) by the non-separation of the anterior and posterior external cusps of the superior molars by an external, rib-like pillar. The next family is the *Chalicotheriidæ*, to which ten genera are referred. The digital formula is the same as in the *Lophiodontidæ*, as is also the relation of the molar and premolar teeth. The only distinction is found in the separation of the anterior and posterior external lobes by a vertical ridge. The remains of this family range from the lower Eocene to the middle Miocene. The third family is the *Palæotheriidæ*, having three toes on each foot. The molars and premolars are alike, and the inferior molars possess perfect double crescents. The fourth family is the *Equidæ*, in which the digital formula is reduced to one toe on each foot. The molars and premolars are alike and highly complex in structure. It is to this family that all the existing horses belong, and it has been traced as far back as the upper Miocene strata. The *Condylarthra*, on the other hand, are effectually separated from the *Perissodactyla* by the non-alternating positions of the carpals and by the possession of an astragalus whose distal face is convex in every direction, as in the carnivora, and unites with the navicular alone. These families are the *Phenacodontidæ* and *Meniscotheriidæ* whose remains have been found so far only in the lower Eocene deposits of this country. It is interesting to note that they are the most generalized of any known Perissodactyla and supply a link long sought in the evolution of the later and more specialized forms of this order.

\* There has probably been no discovery among the ungulates since the finding of the *Amblypoda* that has proved equal in interest and importance to the discovery of this group (the Phenacodontidæ). The descent of all the ungulates from the *Amblypoda* has been held by Prof. Cope for some time, but that it took place from any *known* genera of this order the comparatively specialized condition of the teeth of the latter distinctly forbids. This moderate complexity of the teeth among Eocene mammals is a striking exception, especially when associated with such a low grade of organization of other parts as we find in these animals. The explanation of this fact must, in my judgment, be sought for in their large size and in the possession of powerful canine teeth, which insure them greater immunity from the attacks of fierce carnivorous contemporaries. With these means of defense, they could take up their abode where food better adapted to their wants was furnished. Hence we can with perfect consistency look for a rapid modification of these organs, accompanied by slight change in others. In order to make the connection complete between them and the Phenacodonts, there should yet be found an Amblypod with bunodont

3—3; canines, 1—1, 1—1; premolars, 4—4, 4—4; molars, 3—3, 3—3 = 44; that is 44 functionally developed teeth. The molars are of the simple four-lobed pattern, resembling in this respect the suilline Artiodactyla or hogs and peccaries; in fact on this account it is a matter of some surprise that the animal should

molars, reduced canines and a more elongated foot. An approach to this condition, as far at least as the molars are concerned, is found in a new form recently described by Prof. Cope under the name Manteodon (prophecy tooth). The *Amblypoda*, says Prof. Cope in his Report on Capt. Wheeler's Survey (W. 100th Mer., Pt. ii, Vol. IV, p. 233), are as yet confined to the Eocene period exclusively, and are found both in Europe and this country. In points of affinity to the hoofed orders generally they occupy an interesting and important position, being in all probability the oldest and affording the most generalized condition known among the ungulates. The brain capacity is exceedingly small in proportion to the size of the other parts of the skeleton, and from casts made from the brain case itself we are warranted in assigning these animals a position among the lowest mammalia; they are lower in brain development even than any of the *Marsupials*. The feet are very short, are provided with five fully developed toes, and have their entire plantar and palmar surfaces applied to the ground, as in the modern bears. The astragalus is greatly flattened from above downward, and is primitive and characteristic. It displays on its inferior surface flattened articular facets for both navicular and cuboid bones which share the articulation about equally. On the superior part, the surface articulating with the tibia is almost flat, a condition which must have rendered the ankle joint capable of very little movement, and giving to these animals a peculiarly awkward and shambling gait. It is not difficult to perceive that these small-brained, five-toed, and plantigrade *Amblypoda* could easily have furnished a starting point for both the *Artiodactyla* and *Perissodactyla*, and, as we have good reasons to believe, did give origin to the *Proboscidea* or elephants.

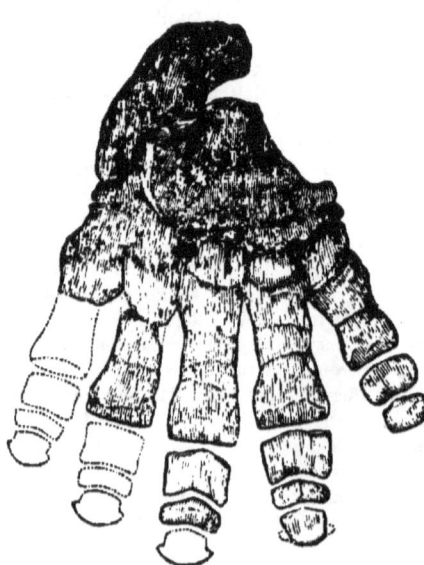

Right hind-foot of a species of Coryphodon (Amblypod), half natural size (Cope).

turn out not to belong to the suillines. But when the evidence of derivation drawn from other sources is considered, and the geological period is taken into account, the structure of the teeth is preëminently in accordance with the expectations of the evolutionist. It is important to notice in this connection that Prof. Cope ventured the prediction in 1874[*] that the quadritubercular or four-lobed bunodont [†] molar was the primitive pattern in which the more complicated selenodont [‡] molar of the later ungulates had its origin. That this prediction is now proved there can be no question, and the passage from this simple type of tooth to the highly complicated forms illustrated in this article has, I think, been close and consecutive and intimately associated with reduction in digits.

The Phenacodontidæ present considerable variety as far as their family is at present known. Prof. Cope has described five genera, as follows: Phenacodus, Anacodon, Protogonia, Periptychus, and Anisonchus. The first two are from the Wasatch horizon, while the last three were derived from the underlying Puerco beds. Periptychus shows a peculiar sculpturing of the outside of the molar teeth, similar to that seen in many reptiles, and is the only mammal known to possess it. The molars of Anacodon lack distinct tubercles, a character which assigns it the lowest position in the family. Phenacodus approaches nearest to the Lophiodons in dental character and is taken for illustration. As all but Phenacodus and Periptychus are known from their teeth only, it may be necessary on the discovery of the character of their feet to refer them to new families. The definition of the family given by Prof. Cope is as follows: Molar teeth tubercular; molars and premolars different; five toes on all the feet.[§]

### MENISCOTHERIUM.

The Meniscotheriidæ has been recently established for the reception of the single genus Meniscotherium, discovered by

---

[*] Journal Academy of Natural Sciences, Philadelphia.
[†] Teeth of simple structure, with short crowns and low, blunt tubercles on their face.
[‡] Teeth of complicated structure, with high and uniformly broadened crowns, the face presenting a complex folding of the enamel plates.
[§] Palæontological Bulletin, No. 34, Dec., 1881, p. 173.

Prof. Cope in the Wasatch beds of New Mexico, and described by him in his report to Captain Wheeler, already cited. It was formerly arranged in the *Chalicotheriidæ*, near *Chalicotherium*, with which it agrees in all essential dental characters. The recent discovery of the bones of the feet shows that they display the characteristic peculiarities of the *Condylarthra*, to which group it must be referred. Its digital formula is unknown, hence we must rely on the specialized crescentoid pattern of the molars for the family definition. It is proper to remark here that reduction in digits in the Perissodactyla is usually accompanied by specialization of the molar teeth. In this case, therefore, I would venture the prediction that its digital formula will be found to be 4—3, with the outer toes somewhat reduced. The value of the digital formula as a character in the definition of the families of the Perissodactyla is of high standard. This may likewise be said of the relation of the molar and premolar teeth, but in a less degree. The tubercular or crescentoid structure of the molars, however, is capable of such intergradation, which increase of our knowledge demonstrates, that it must be accepted as provisional only, and not entitled to rank equal in value to either of the other two characters in defining the family.

The genealogy of the horse as now indicated is as follows:

PERISSODACTYLA - { Equus,            Equus,
                                Protohippus,      Hippotherium,
                                 Anchippus, Paloplotherium,
                                   Anchitherium,
                                   Mesohippus,
                                   Lambdotherium,
                                   Hyracotherium,
                                   Systemodon.

AMBLYPODA,                   Hyodonta (Cope).

CONDYLARTHRA - { Meniscotherium,
                               Phenacodus.

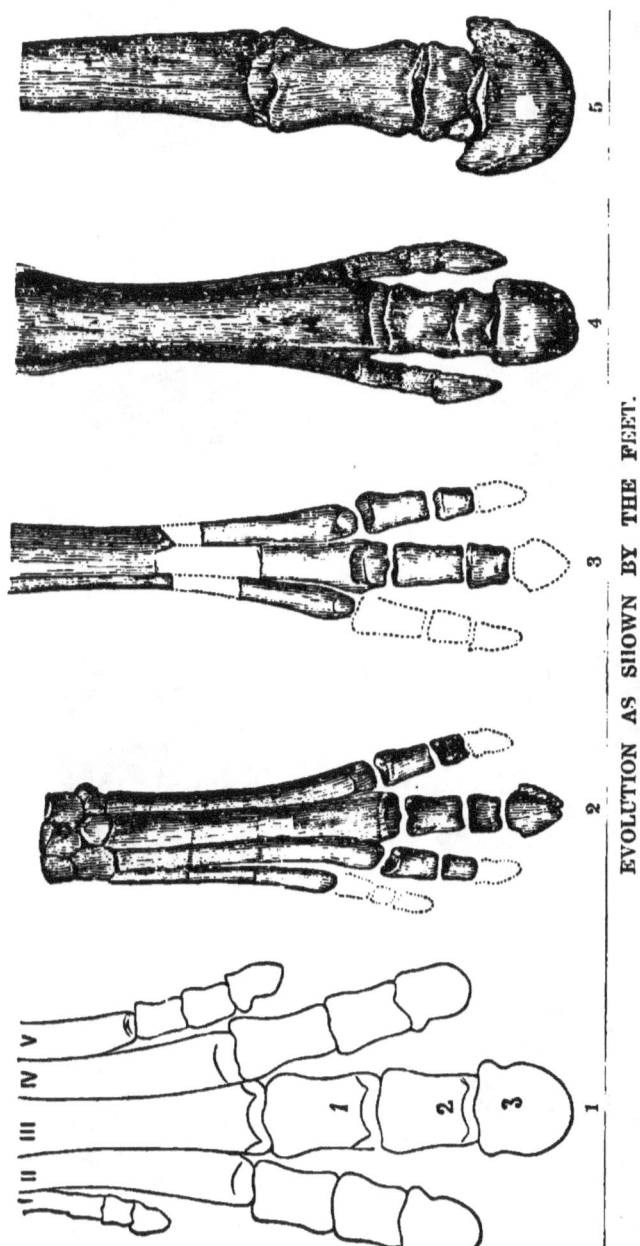

EVOLUTION AS SHOWN BY THE FEET.

1. Left hind foot of *Phenacodus primaevus*; half natural size (Cope). 2. Left fore foot of *Hyracotherium venticolum*; half natural size (Wortman). 3. Hind foot of same, a reduction of one toe from the fore and two from the hind foot. 4. Left fore foot of *Anchitherium aurelianense*; one-fifth natural size (Gaudry). 5. Left fore foot of *Equus caballus* (modern horse); one-fifth natural size (Gaudry).

266    APPENDIX.

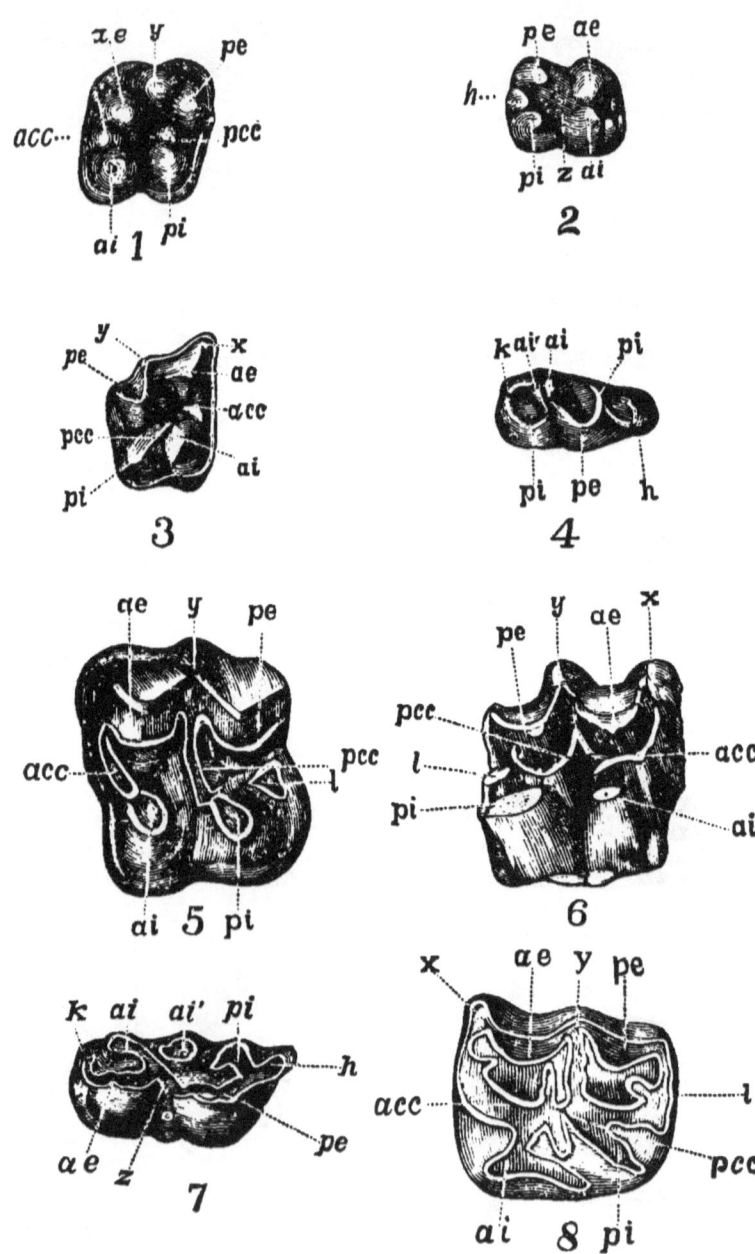

1.—Left upper molar of a species of *Phenacodus*, nat. size (Cope) *ae* is the antero-external, *pe* the postero-external, *ai* the antero-internal and *pi* the postero-internal lobes respectively. They are low and obtuse and constitute the principal cusps of the crown. *acc* and *pcc* are the anterior and posterior cross crests; they are rudimentary and represented by isolated tubercles in this animal, but are developed into important structures in the more specialized genera. *y* (the lobe is drawn too large) is the rudimental external rib separating the antero and postero-external cusps. An antero-basal lobe arising as an outgrowth from the cingulum or ledge surrounding the base of the crown is strongly marked in some genera.

2.—Left lower molar of same, nat. size. *z* represents a low, indistinctly marked ridge, passing from the postero-external to the antero-internal cusps *pe*, *ai*. The antero-internal cusp *ai* is sometimes double. *h* is the heel, which is so strong in the last molar as to be called a fifth lobe. It is connected by a faint ridge with the postero-external cusp *pe*. The four principal cusps *ae*, *pe*, *ai*, *pi* hold the same relation to the crown as in the upper molar.

3.—Right upper molar, of a species of *Lambdotherium*, in which the antero and postero-external cusps *ae*, *pe* are separated by an external vertical ridge, *y* ; nat. size (Cope).

4.—Last lower molar (left side), of same ; nat. size. The antero-internal lobe is divided into two distinct tubercles, *ai*, *ai'*; the ridge *k* is strong and prominent. The breadth of the tooth is accounted for by the fact that it is the last molar, the first and last molars being about a third broader than the others. The teeth are of a more complicated pattern than those of Phenacodus. It is important to notice that while the teeth of the lower Eocene genera of this family (Lambdotherium and Palæosyopous) resemble very strongly the teeth of the lower forms of the Lophiodons in the shortness of their crowns and approach to the bunodont type, the latter possess longer cusps and simulate the selenodont forms in the crescentic section of some of them.

5.—Left upper molar of *Anchitherium aureliquense*, nat. size (Gaudry). The four principal cusps *ae*, *pe*, *ai*, *pi* are considerably lengthened and connected by high ridges, *acc*, *pcc*, which pass in an oblique direction across the crown. The elevation of the cusps and crests give increased depth to the valleys. The anterior basal lobe is reduced and the external rib *y* is strong. The crown is further complicated by the addition of the lobe *l*.

6.—Right upper molar of a species of *Hippotherium*. The valleys, which are deepened by the lengthening of the cusps and ridges, are filled by a thick deposit of cement, but the cement, as the cut shows, has been removed. The points of the cusps and ridges are unworn. The four principal lobes *ae*, *pe*, *ai*, *pi* hold about the same relation to each other. The cross crests *acc*, *pcc* have their obliquities increased, and the anterior bends around on the inner part of the face and becomes confluent with the posterior ridge *pcc*. The lobe *l*, which is conic in Anchitherium, is elongated in a transverse direction to the crown, so as to close the posterior valley and join the posterior external cusp *pe* with the posterior crest *pcc*. Additional vertical pillars are developed on the cross ridges. The teeth resem-

7.—Left lower molar of *Hippotherium gracile*, three-fourths natural size (Gaudry). The lobe $ai'$ is now completely separated and the ridge $k$ rises to a level with the other cusps. The heel $h$ is also elevated and connected by a strong ridge. The filling up of the valleys by a deposit of cementum and the consequent attrition in mastication produce a marked change in appearance from that seen in Anchitherium, but by close observation the strictest homology is seen to exist.

8.—Left upper molar of a species of *Equus* (modern horse) natural size. The internal lobes $ai$, $pi$ are connected with the cross ridges $acc$, $pcc$. The only difference of generic value between *Equus* and *Hippidium* (a near relative of the horse) is seen in the relative size of the antero and postero-internal lobes $ai$, $pi$; in Equus $ai$ is greatly enlarged and somewhat flattened; in Hippidium the lobes are almost equal.

What has caused these changes? In regard to tooth structure generally, Mr. J. A. Ryder has given us a most excellent treatise "On the Mechanical Genesis of Tooth Forms,"* in which he shows that the jaw movements of animals are intimately related to the modification of the component lobes, crests, and ridges of the crowns of the molar teeth. He also points out that the restricted jaw movements, in which the mouth is simply opened and closed, are associated with the bunodont molar; that the various kinds of excursive mandibular movements have been developed progressively; "that as these movements have increased in complexity there has been increase in the complexity of the enamel foldings."

If we attempt to apply these facts to the ancestry of the horse, it is by no means difficult to perceive that gradual change of habitat, causing a corresponding change in diet, would also compel greater and greater mobility of the mandibular articulation for proper trituration of the new food. The movements of the lower jaw in these animals have assumed a lateral direction, which affords, as I believe, a sufficient explanation for the broadening of the crowns and the lateral flattening of the cusps. The obvious effect of force continually applied in this direction would be to wrinkle the enamel covering of the cusps and ridges, thereby producing the accessory pillars seen in the higher types. By this method, I believe, a more and more complex grinding surface has been produced.

* Proceedings Academy Natural Sciences, Philadelphia, 1878.

The cause of digital reduction is another interesting inquiry. Bunodonts as a rule are dwellers in swamps and forests and live on nuts, berries, and roots. If they are compelled to forsake their natural habitat and live in the open field, either modification or extinction will follow. Once in the open field speed becomes a desideratum as a condition of safety, and the foot with a reduced number of digits possesses many advantages over the polydactyle one.

Prof. Cope has shown (*American Naturalist*, April, 1881) that in plantigrade quadrupeds the extremities of the toes are arranged in a semicircle, when they are all applied to the ground. In the act of running the heel and wrist are raised, throwing the weight of the body on the median digits. An infinite repetition of this posture in digitigrade animals unable to withstand the attacks of their enemies and whose only escape was in flight, the strengthening of the median digits, and the consequent reduction of the outer ones, would follow according to the law of use and disuse of parts. This subtraction of toes has progressed step by step until the modern one-toed horse has been reached.

In summing up an article in the *Kansas City Review of Science and Industry*, Mr. Wortman says:

"I dare say that if all the intervening individuals between Phenacodus and Equus could be produced classification would be utterly impossible, so insensible would be the gradation."

The forms already known appear to point to the inevitable conclusion that the modern horse is the product of the slow but improving processes of evolution, which are still in operation, and are being aided by all the skill known to modern science. A discussion of the subject is almost superfluous, for the illustrations, like deeds, speak louder than words.

*Note.*—Pliny (B.C. 23) says Cæsar had a 5-toed horse (the forefeet), which was represented in his (Pliny's) day by a statue; also that Epigenes says the Babylonians had a series of observations on the stars for a period of 720,000 years, inscribed on *baked bricks*. Berosus and Critodemus say 490,000. (Vol. ii. pp. 221-317.) Baked bricks have been found buried in the valley of the Nile at a depth to require the annual deposits of that river for 9,000 years (72 feet.) May they not some day be valuable aids to science as well as history? Their stories can be better imagined than described

## THE VIEWS OF AN EVOLUTIONIST.

The following "review" of Horses' Teeth, written by Mr. R. M. Tuttle for *Johnstons' Dental Miscellany*, contains so much of interest on the subject of evolution that I think no apology necessary for inserting it here instead of putting it among the other press reviews at the conclusion of the volume:

"The author of this work modestly suggests that it may be of value to the veterinary profession and also to horsemen and farmers. We have no hesitation in going further and affirming that it contains much of an instructive and interesting character for dentists, and all scientific and thoughtful men. The day has gone by when humanity laughed or grew angry (according to its temper at the moment) at the mere suggestion that man has any relationship with the lower animals beyond their submission to his will and his right to lead them to the slaughter-house. The movement of thought in the direction of Evolution is battled against by some eminent thinkers. The book before us does much to upset the arguments of these thinkers and to support the theory they denounce. But there is a middle position for those who neither agree with the theory of a separate creation for every genus nor with the development of animal life from one germ form. This position may be described in the words of Tennyson as a 'sunless gulf of doubt.' Doubt, however, is not always sunless; and besides to admit a doubt is at least frank, and we prefer it to being dogmatic. Still even believers in a separate creation for every genus cannot but admit that, notwithstanding the great diversity in the animal kingdom, there is a oneness of principle, a common style of architecture, so to speak, pervading all animal life, which we see in the structure of teeth, arms, legs, wings, &c.

"The construction of a horse's teeth points to the inevitable conclusion that he is a vegetarian, but the various changes in the dentition of a long line of fossil horses indicate that he was once probably carnivorous, or perhaps omnivorous. Teeth, like other parts of the body, are influenced by use; the change is not so obvious, but it is no less certain. As the volume before us affirms, for example, the canine and remnant teeth have been much reduced in size, and, if Mr. Darwin's theory is correct, are probably in the course of ultimate extinction. Now, the function of a canine tooth is to tear, not grind. If animals that now use their canines for tearing flesh were compelled to subsist on vegetable food, there would perhaps be no marked change in a generation, but there certainly would be in a series of generations. We therefore conclude that horse dentures have adapted themselves to a gradual but great change in the animal's mode of existence, a gradual departure from the original custom of subsisting on food which demanded tearing teeth, and that it took to vegetarianism naturally. Fossil remains would force this conclusion on us, however much we might desire to doubt it. But why should we have such a desire? To admit development, say some, is but the thin end of the wedge of Evolution. Be it so. It is the function of scientific wedges to split old and false notions, and who ever heard of a man putting the thick end of a wedge in first? Whether development is the thin end of the wedge of Evolution or not we do not care much to inquire. If a man studies horses' teeth of to-day as well as those of human beings, he will come to the conclusion that in both there are signs of great development when compared with the teeth of thousands of years ago. He will observe not change merely, but signs of a *higher order of being*—signs of an evolution of the *superior* from the *inferior*.

"To some people Evolution is a bugbear, and the idea that human beings are capable of physical development is not much less. We advise such people not to read Mr. Clarke's book. It would trouble them. They might cast it into the fire and thus waste their money. But intelligent seekers after truth, those who find the 'gulf of doubt' in which they are floundering too sunless for their light-loving souls; those who are not afraid to meet the doctrines of scientific men face to face, may read this work with profit. Without desiring to disparage its author, we may say that its chief value lies in the fact that it is composed largely of selections from the works of men of special knowledge on the subject of the treatise and of various germain subjects. Much credit is due to him for collecting in so compact a form such a large quantity of valuable matter, which was scattered over cyclopedias, translations of learned societies, and other costly books."

Mr. Tuttle, in a letter to me (a few words of which have been interpolated in the foregoing article), in substance says:

"At the close of the Eocene period there were three distinct types of animals descended from a common ancestor that are now represented by the horse, tapir, and rhinoceros.* Let us suppose that a pair of animals gave birth to the offspring which were to be the parents of these three types. What would be the process of development? These animals, with their mates, by some means get separated. The parent of the future tapir goes one way; that of the rhinoceros stays at home, while he who is to beget the horse wanders away from the marshes and rivers to the dryer land. Circumstances over which he has no adequate control place him where alligators, crocodiles, and other animals that he has been accustomed to attack with his tushes are absent. His feet, which are many-toed, broad, and adapted to walking in the mud, now tread hard soil; his canine teeth, which were used in tearing flesh, now find little employment; his neck, from constant stretching as he crops the foliage of the bushes, lengthens; a more rapid gait is acquired by a gradual contraction of the toes and the lengthening of the legs, and eventually this modified animal becomes a horse. Thus is told in a few words what I believe has been going on in the course of hundreds of thousands, perhaps millions of years."

It is noteworthy that a young man like Mr. Tuttle should entertain views similar to those of such an experienced evolutionist as Prof. Cope. It is not difficult to believe that the bear-like Amblypoda, which Prof. Cope thinks were the common progenitors of the horse, tapir, rhinoceros, elephant, &c., were carnivorous, and there certainly is some analogy between the supposititious animal just described by Mr. Tuttle and the Amblypoda. Change of food was probably as instrumental in producing the great physical changes in early fossil animals as change of habitat and climate. And change of food does not

---

\* Compare with quotation from Prof. Huxley in third note, pp. 65-66; also with same from Prof. Owen, pp. 106-7.

necessarily entail extinction, unless it be food directly opposed to the animal's nature ; and it matters not if the change *is* compulsory, for changes of taste may be either natural or cultivated. For example, children relish food they cannot eat when adult, and *vice versâ*, which is natural ; and an appetite for some foods may be cultivated at any age. Again, food probably causes much of the change in tame boars and other animals that become wild, and *vice versâ*. Still it is not strictly correct to say that the horse *as such* was ever carnivorous, for an animal that was the common ancestor of so many diverse animals was as much one as the other.

In 1878, in a hastily written prospectus of a work that Dr. C. D. House designed to publish, in conformity with his (House's) views, I said the horse was probably once carnivorous. Thinking Dr. House to be mistaken, I wrote to Dr. Leidy of Philadelphia, asking his opinion on the subject. He agreed with me.

## THE ORIGINAL HOME OF THE HORSE.

THERE is no doubt that the original home of the horse is not Europe, but Central Asia ; for since the horse in its natural state depends on grass for its nourishment and fleetness for its weapon (safety), it could not in the beginning have thriven and multiplied in the thick forest-grown territory of Europe. Much rather should its place of propagation be sought in those steppes where it still roams about in a wild state. Here too arose the first nations of riders of which we have historic knowledge, the Mongolians and the Turks, whose existence, even at this day, is as it were combined with that of the horse. From these regions the horse spread in all directions, especially into the steppes of Southern and Southeastern Russia and into Thrace, until it finally found entrance into the other parts of Europe, but not until after the immigration of the people. This assumption is at least strongly favored by the fact that the further a district of Europe is from those Asiatic steppes, *i. e.*, from the original home of the horse, the later does the tamed horse seem to have made its historic appearance in it. The supposition is further confirmed by the fact that horse-raising among almost every tribe appears as an art derived from neighboring tribes in the East or Northeast. Even in Homer the ox appears exclusively as the draught-animal in land operations at home and in the field, while the horse was used for purposes of war only. Its employment in military operations was determined by swiftness alone. That the value of the horse must originally have depended on its fleetness, can easily be inferred from the name that is repeated in all the branches of the Indo-European language, and signifies nearly "hastening," "quick." The same fact is exemplified by the descriptions of the oldest poets, who, next to its courage, speak most of its swiftness.—*The Popular Science Monthly for June, 1882.*

## ELEPHANT TOOTH-GERMS.

MM. POUCHET AND CHABRIT *(Le Progrès Médical)*, having examined the germs of the teeth of a fetus of an elephant in the *Jardin des Plantes*, have concluded that the general opinions on this subject are not exact. Since the works of Robin and Kölliker, it has been assumed that there is produced on the surface of the gum a primary epithelial bud (bourgeon), that Pouchet calls the epithelial plate and Kölliker the adamantine organ or enamel, which sends out a prolongation destined to form a temporary tooth, and afterward a second prolongation for a permanent tooth. The more recent experiments seem to prove that the permanent teeth are not given forth from the neck of the temporary, and that there is no secondary adamantine organ. In the elephant, where there is no second set of teeth, the same plate or layer appears, together with the same prolongations. The two faces of the epithelial prolongation do not have the same structure; the inner face is composed of cylindrical cells, while in the outer face there is a mingling of epithelial and tissue cells.—*N. Y. Med. Times, Feb. 1881 (translated by Dr. T. M. Strong).*

The deductions of MM. Pouchet and Chabrit may be correct in principle, but it is a mistake to say the elephant has only one set of teeth, for he has six or more, and may in fact be said to be always teething. The following facts are partly based on Cuvier, Owen, and Wm. Jacobs:

The grinders, which are constantly in progress of destruction and formation, are not deciduous in the ordinary sense, for they succeed each other horizontally instead of vertically, and not more than one wholly or two partially (one on each side in each jaw) is in use at one time. As the fore part of the tooth in use is worn away by attrition and its roots diminished by absorption, its successor pushes it forward (a movement that appears to be facilitated by the direct backward and forward action of the lower jaw), and a large part of the replacing tooth is in use for some time before the first is entirely shed. Thus a grinding surface is ready all the time. The milk teeth are cut eight or ten days after birth, the upper preceding the lower, and it is about two years before they are entirely displaced by the second set. The second set is in use, but gradually disappearing, from the second year to the sixth, when the third is fully in position; it in turn serves till the ninth year, when the fourth set is in position; and thus it continues to the end of the animal's life—100 or even 150 years. Each succeeding tooth requires at least a year more than its predecessor to be completed.

The grinders are remarkable for their size and the complexity of their structure, the upper and lower teeth being much alike. They are composed of ivory (dentine), enamel, and a large quantity of cement. The crown is short in proportion to the depth of the base or root, only a small part appearing above the gum. In the Asiatic species the crown is composed of transverse, vertical, enamel-plated dentine ridges, about half an inch apart, and joined together by cement. The ridges are nearly straight and are tooth-like in appearance. The ridges are good indicators of age, the first set of teeth having 4, the second 8 or 9, the third 12 or 13, the fourth 15, and so on to the seventh or eighth, which have 22 or 23. In the African species the crown is studded by lozenge-shaped projections instead of ridges. A tooth of the elephant *Columbus*, an excellent specimen, which may be seen in Worth's Museum (New York), weighs 12 pounds; its breadth is 7 inches (the aggregate of the six back teeth of the horse); thickness, $2\frac{1}{2}$; length, 11.

It has only 13 crown ridges, and is therefore little above a medium-sized tooth.* The crown resembles a small Belgian paving stone, while the taper of the root resembles that of a heart.

The elephant is a vegetarian, and the construction of its grinders is a striking example of the adaptation of the teeth of an animal to its food.

The tusks, two in number and belonging to the upper jaw, are shed but once. The deciduous tusks cut between the fifth and seventh months and are shed about the end of the first year, their roots being considerably absorbed. They rarely exceed 2 inches in length and ⅜ of an inch in diameter. About two months after the shedding of the temporary tusks, the permanent, which are situated to the inner side of and behind the former, emerge and continue to grow throughout life. They have an enamel coat, but are mostly composed of ivory, a remarkably fine and elastic form of dentine (differing somewhat from the dentine of other teeth), and are hollow for a considerable part of their length. They are deeply imbedded in the skull. Sir Samuel Baker found one 8 feet long with 22 inches girth to be imbedded 31 inches.

The tusks, which are formidable defensive and offensive weapons, and which correspond to the canine teeth of other animals, vary much in length, weight, and curvature. Gordon Cumming found a tusk in Africa that measured 10¾ feet and weighed 173 pounds. The average, however, is not over 7 feet and 100 pounds. They are generally smaller in the female than in the male, but according to Cuvier the African species are the same in this respect. In the Indian elephant some have a pronounced upward curve, some are nearly straight, while others resemble the letter S. They are sometimes used as levers in uprooting mimosa trees whose crown of foliage is beyond the reach of the trunk. In Ceylon, where the elephant lives chiefly on grass and herbage, the tusks are generally absent in both sexes. The bullets sometimes found in the ivory are probably first lodged in the pulp cavity and then carried to the solid part by growth.

---

\* Mr. L. G. Yates of Centerville, California, says fossil elephant molars weighing 25 pounds have been discovered in that State.

A large elephant weighs 7,000 pounds. The Indian elephant is 10 feet in hight, the African 12; a skeleton in the St. Petersburg Museum is 16½.

---

## HUMAN TEETH.

### FILLING CHILDREN'S TEETH.*

FILLING the deciduous or first set of teeth prevents decay and consequent injury to the second set,† alleviates pain, facilitates speech,‡ mastication, and regularity in the growth of the second set, aids in keeping the breath pure, and is conducive to health at a very critical time of life. They should be filled as long as filling will preserve their usefulness, and at all times, for some are shed as early as the fifth or sixth year, others as late as the eleventh or twelfth. Any of the usual fillings will answer, the sole object being to arrest decay and "aid somatic development" (Odell). Children should be taught to use a brush and proper dentifrices. Defective teeth are often the result of improper diet during utro-gestation. Drs. J. Allen and G. M. Eddy say that mothers do not eat enough bone-producing food, such as oatmeal, bread made from unbolted flour, &c., but admit that such foods do not assimilate in every case. Dentists differ as to the advisability of the use of anæsthetics in treating children.

The teething period is longer than is usually supposed. It begins about the seventh month before birth§ and continues

---

\* The object of this brief article is merely to call attention to an important subject. My own attention was directed to it by Mr. E. A. Rockwell in an interesting article in the *New York Sun*. Readers who wish to study the subject are referred to the elaborate works of dentists. Besides the dentists mentioned above I have consulted Drs. G. H. Rich, F. Abbott, and C. E. and J. S. Latimer, all of New York.

† Dr. T. P. Wagoner (Knightstown, Ind., *Dental News*) approves the above, and in addition says the development of a permanent tooth may be retarded by a dead deciduous tooth.

‡ Haller and other physiologists give minute accounts of the effects produced by teeth in articulating the various letters of the alphabet.—*Bostock*.

§ For the development of human tooth-germs from the seventh week till birth see page 46.

till the age of 17 or 25 years. The annexed cut (Farrar) represents (above the dotted line) an upper deciduous set of teeth. 1, 1, central incisors, erupt between the 5th and 6th months; 2, 2, lateral incisors, 7th and 10th months; 3, 3, canines (eye teeth), 12th and 16th months; 4, 4, 5, 5, all molars, 14th and 36th months. Total, 20. The lower teeth usually precede the upper by a few weeks. 6, 6 do not belong to the deciduous set, but, as they erupt between the fifth and sixth years, are usually classed with them, and frequently decay beyond remedy before the mistake is discovered.

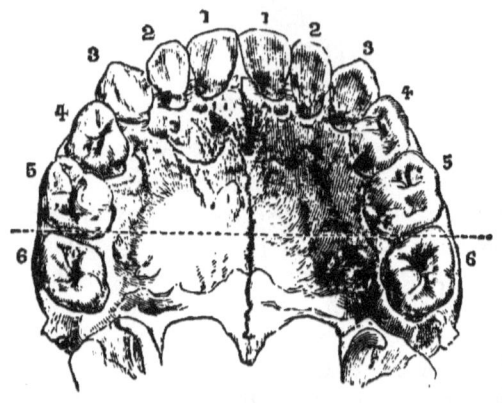

Dr. J. N. Farrar (New York), to whose works I am indebted for information, says (*Missouri Dental Journal*, April, 1880): "The statistics in this country show that out of about 80 people of all classes only one has sound teeth. This is the result of a combination of causes—systemic disturbances from climate, food, crossing of races and types, and neglect. Most of the cavities are caused by anatomical imperfections or overcrowding, nearly all of which develop before the thirty-fifth year. * * * The science of dentistry, however, has checked much of this suffering, and at this time (1879) there are 12,000 dentists annually packing into tooth-cavities about half a ton of gold—$500,000. The estimated gold coinage value in this country is about $150,000,000; this sum, at the rate gold is used for fillings, would be transferred to graveyards in 300 years. The value of the cheap fillings is about $100,000, and there are annually manufactured about 3,000,000 artificial (porcelain) teeth. * * * If $100 is put on interest (7 per cent.) at the birth of a child, it ought to pay all dental expenses till the age of 30 years; but if the child's teeth are neglected, increased dental bills result, with poor teeth at best. The only question remaining is, is the baby worth $100?"

# INDEX.

ABNORMAL DENTITION, human, 128; horse, 142.
Abnormal Teeth, 115-123.
Abnormal Tooth, description of, 123.
Absorption of roots of foals' teeth, 48, 70-1; do. elephant, 275-6; dental journal on, 288.
Alfort Veterinary College, 14), 142.
Amblypoda, the, 257; description of, 261-2.
Americas, the, richness of fossil remains in, 10)-113.
Anacodon, fossil horse, 263.
Anchippus, fossil horse, 95.
Anchitherium, fossil horse, 96, 111.
Anchitherium aureliauense, teeth of, 236-7; toes of, 263.
Animal Kingdom, diversity yet oneness of principle in, 270.
Animal, a supposititious, 272.
Anoplothere, teeth of, 65.
Antelope montana, tushes of, 78.
Apparatus, dental, exuberance of particular parts of, 141-3.
Appendix, fossil horses, evolution, original home of horse, elephant and children's teeth, 257-277.
Apsyrtus, advice of, 116.
Arcades (of teeth) anomalies in form of, 140, 141.
Aristotle, mistake of, 69.
Arloing, M., resection of nerves, 217.
Armadillo, the, 229.
Artiodactyla (hogs, &c.), 257, 262.
Ass, experiment on an, 217, 218.

BABINGTON, B., 242.
Bacon, Francis, theory of, 15.
Baer, Von, comparisons by, 81.
Baker, S., report of, 181, 182.
Batrachia, the, 229, 230.
Bay, Surgeon, discovery of, 117.
Bell, C., discoveries of, 217, 218.
Bell, Thomas, theories of, 26-7, 83-4.
Berger-Perriere, discovery of, 116.
Berzelius, discoveries of, 15.

Birds, fossil, teeth of, 114.
'Bishoping,' modus operandi of, 211.
Black, Surgeon, experiment of, 29.
Blaine, Surgeon, fractured jaw, 197.
Blastema, nature and color of, 84-5.
Blumenbach, on quadrumana, 251.
Boar, the masked, grinders of, 10.
Boar, wild, tame, changes in, 81, 273.
Boll, Dr., tooth pulp, 51.
Bojanus, discovery of, 52.
Bond's 'Dental Medicine,' extract from, 128, 129.
Bouley, M. H., development of teeth, 45; grinders, 62; formation of enamel, 64; growth of teeth during life, 73; diseases of teeth, 128; diseases and dentistry of teeth, 129-162; swallowing teeth, 192, 193; removal of fractured jaw, 197, 198.
Bourgelat, Prof., milk molars, 69.
Brandt, L., length of incisors, 74; age of Spanish horses, crib-biters and mules, 215; age by shape of teeth, 215.
Brewster, B. S., letter from, 292.
Broadhead, G. C., account of fossil tooth, 112, 113.
Broderip, Mr., a whale's tooth, 79.
Burns, John, description by, 239.
Butterfly, the, transformations of, 81.

CACHALOT, the, 79.
Calcigerous, origin of word, 18.
Cattle, teething period of, 91, 92.
Camel, the, teeth of, 66.
Camper, P., temporary canines, 52.
Canines, temporary, 51, 52.
Calculus Concretions, 192, 193, 230.
Caries, cause of, 144-154; 165-173; symptoms of, 148-154; different in different teeth, 151; odor of, 153; treatment of, 155-171; treatment after trephining sinuses for, 176; other dental cases, 177-193; confounded with glanders, 176, 180, 183; definition of, 231.

Cartwright, W. A., report of, 193; fracture of jawbone, 196.
Caucasian Races, teeth of, 99.
Cement, the, 9; size of tubes of, 16; use of, 17; mistaken for tartar, 17; vascularity of, 17; thinness of, 17; color of, 18; resemblance to bone, 23; germs of, 43; a protecting varnish, 59, 60; microscopical character of, 133.
Chabrit, M., tooth-germs, 274.
Challcotheriidæ (fossil horses), 260.
Chandler, C. F., on albumen, 227.
Chauveau, A., harmony of teeth with general system, 11; development of tooth-germs, 41, 42; description of incisors, 58, 59, 60; growth of teeth during life, 73.
Cherry, W. A., shedding teeth, 50-1; judging age by shape of teeth, 204.
Chevrotain, 78; description of, 232.
Clayworth, Surg., report of, 197.
Coleman, Surgeon, discovery of, 116.
'Columbus' (elephant), tooth of, 275.
Coluber Scaber (serpent), 121.
Comparative Anatomy, 233.
Conrad, T., discovery of, 113.
Complex grinders, cause of, 268.
Concomitant Variation, a factor in evolution problem, 98.
Condylarthra, the, 260-1, 264.
Cope, E. D., editor American Naturalist, 113; physiological homologies, 248; discovers Phenacodus (teeth) and other fossil horses, 259-269; opinion of the Amblypoda, 261-2.
Copybara, the, grinders of, 10; description of, 230.
Coughing and Teething, treatment for, 92.
Crib-biting, effect of on teeth, 212-13
Cumming, G., elephant tusk, 276.
Cuvier, F, 13; note on, 65; bones and teeth of recent and fossil horses, 106; ophthalmic ganglion, 221; elephant teeth, 275.

DANA, Prof., geology, 240.
Dandini, J., silver and golden hued teeth, 25-6.
D'Arboval, teething, 87.
Darwin, C. R., tushes of various animals, 77, 78. 79; changes in human teeth, 99.
Dawson, J. W., geology, 240; miocene period, 244; pliocene period, 250.
Day, E. C. H., narwhal, 246.
Deciduous teeth, retention of, 129.
Delafond, M., on trephining, 161.
Denenbourg, F., report of, 133.
Dental Cysts, importance of study of, 115; microscopical character of teeth in, 118; reports and theories on, 115-126.
Dental Canal, the, 31, 224, 234.
Dental Cysts, 115-126.
Dental Nerve, the, 224-226.
Dentinal, origin and use of word, 8.
Dentinal Pulp, network of looped capillaries of the, 33-4.
Dentinal Star, 59; description of, 209.
Dentinal Tubes, office and color of, 22, 23; their two curvatures, 23; dichotomously branched, 131, 133; diameter of, 132; length of curves, 133.
Dentine, the, 8, 14.
Dentine Germ, 43, 59.
Dentition Fever, 93.
Dentition, permanent, 53-74.
Dentition, temporary, 47-52.
Dentition, third, cases of, 128.
Digital reduction, cause of, 269.
Dinoceras mirabilis (fossil), horns and canine teeth of, 236.
Diverticula, use of, 22, 235.
Dog tooth-germs, grafting of, 27-8.
Draper, J. W., obligation to, 4.
Dugong, the, 79; description of, 235.
Dunglison, R., development of teeth, 45; diseases of teeth, 137; calculi, 193; vocabulary, 227-256.

EDDY, Dr., children's teeth, 277.
Edinburgh Veterinary College, report of, 179, 180.
Editor Veterinarian, comments of, 184; report of, 201, 202.
Elasmothere, the, great size of, 107; enamel festoons of molars of, 107; connecting link between horse and rhinoceros, 107.
Elephant, great quantity of cement in grinders of, 10; unique mode of cutting and shedding several dentitions; size, structure, &c., 274-7; affinities with rodents, 200.
Embryo, human, transformations of, 81-2; definition of, 236.
Embryology, 80-82.
Enamel, the, 10; tubes of, 18, 19; color of, 19; membranous sheaths of, 59; plications of, 106.
Enamel, the two rings of, 59.
Enamel-Fibers, direction of, 20; curves of, 20; form and size of, 20; diameter of, 134.
Eocene (period) fossils of, 236.
Equidæ, the, teeth of, 261.
Evolution, doctrine of 77-9, 98-9, 237; 257-6); from inferior to superior, 271; a bugbear, 271.
Exostoses, 17, 116.

FAENKEL, discoveries of, 15.
Falconio, Surg., discovery of, 118.

# INDEX. 281

Ferguson, P. B., development of teeth, 45; grinders, 62; the formation of enamel, 64; growth of teeth during life, 73; diseases of teeth, 138; diseases and dentistry of horses' teeth, 139-162; swallowing teeth, 192, 193.
Filling children's teeth, 277.
Fleming, G., dental cysts, 115-119; fractured jaw, 195, 196; on glanders, 199.
Food, for foals, 50; for tooth-cough, 92; for unequal wear of grinders, 143; after trephining for caries, 153, 162; for defective teeth, improving skin, fever, convalescence, &c., 163-4; sifting of, 171; changes caused by, 272; bone-producing, 277; sugar for horses, 30.
Forthomme, M., milk canines, 52.
Fossil, cat-like animal, a, 244.
Fossil, definition of, 114.
Fossil, hog-like elephant, with tusks in both jaws, 244.
Fossil Horses, cause of changes in teeth of, 268; do. reduction in toes of, 269. (See Horses, fossil.)
Fossil Horses, recent discoveries of, 257-269.
Fossil Tooth, a diseased, 173.
Fractured Jaws, 194-202.
Fungus Hæmatodes, 173; definition of, 239.

GAMGEE, J., report of, 120-2.
Ganglion, nature of, 220-1, 239.
Garengeot, M., dental key, 156.
Generali, Prof., dental cysts, 116-19.
Geology, definition of, 240.
Gill, T., nature of teeth, 12; dental formula for horse, 101; fossil birds' teeth, 114; teeth from diverticula (marsupials), 235; morphology, 245; quadrumana, 231, 232; teleosts, 254.
Girard, M., age by marks and shape, 206-7; dentinal star, 209.
Glanders, resembles caries of last grinders, 152-3; odor of, 159; may be caused by caries of teeth (absorption of pus), 160; sometimes imaginary, 176, 180, 185; danger from and prevalence of. 199.
Gomphosis (tooth-articulation), 72.
Goodsir, Prof., on tooth-germs, 125.
Gorbaux, Surg., discovery of, 117.
Gowing, T. W., on teeth, 171-72.
Grice, C. C., report of, 123, 124.
Grinders, the 54; tables of, 61; figures formed by, 61; contrasts between, 61, 62; their own whetstones, 63; roots of (S. 70; shedding of, 70, 71; activity of growth and undivided base of, 74.
Grouillé, Mage, dental cysts, 116.

Guanaco, 78; description of, 240.
Gubernaculum Dentis, the, description of, 42.
Gums, shrinkage of the, 72, 74, 172, 181; affected by turgescence, 151; nerves of, 225.
Gurlt, Surg., discovery of, 117.
Gutta-percha as a filling for teeth and sinuses, 164, 177; for children's teeth, 277.

HAECKEL, E. H., embryos, 81-2.
Harris, Prof., 3d dentition, 129.
Hartshorne, H., evolution, 237.
Haschischut ed dab, effect of on teeth, 25.
Haw of the horse's eye (membrana nictitans), description of, importance of, and evil caused by ignorant grooms, 244.
Hayden, Dr., discoveries of, 257.
Hayes, B., tooth-pulp, dentinal tubes, cells and curves upon curves, cement, enamel, &c., 22-4; diseases of teeth. 137.
Heard, J. M., obligation to, 216; letter from, 292.
Heath, J. P., report of, 200, 201.
Hénocque, M., motor nerves, 217.
Herbert, W. H., age, 214, 215.
Hesperornis (bird), teeth of, 114.
Hesperornis regalis, teeth of, 114.
Hipparion, fossil horse, 95, 96, 111.
Hippotherium, fossil horse, 264-7.
Hippotherium gracile, 268.
Hippopotamus, canine teeth of, 63.
Histology, definition of, 241.
Hitchcock, C. H., on fossils, 114.
Hocing, C. F., obligation to, 215; letter from, 292.
Hog, canine teeth of, 63.
Horsburgh, J., report of, 175.
Horse, signification of word, 274.
Horse, the, theory of introduction into America, 110; a vegetarian, 270; probably never carnivorous, 272-3; once used for war only, 274.
Horse Dentistry, argument in favor of, 160; dental and other journals on, 287-292.
Horse, genealogy of, 264.
Horse, original home of, 273.
Horses, fossil, A. acodon, 263; Anchippus, 96, 264; Anchitherium, 96, 111, 112, 264; Anchitherium aurelianense, 265, 267; Anisonchus, 263; Chalicotheriidæ, 260, 264; Eohippus, (suppositious), 259; Equidæ, 261; Equus caballus primigenius, 107; Equus complicatus, 113; Equus curvidens, 107; Equus fossilis, 106; Equus piicidens, 107; Equus primigenius, 107; Hipparion, 95-6, 111, 112; Hippidium, 268; Hippotherium, 264-7;

Hippotherium gracile, 268; Hyodonta, 254; Hyohippus, 112; Hyracotherium, 253, 264-5; Lambdotherium, 264-7; Lophiodon and Lophiodontide, 258, 259; Meniscotherium, 263-4; Merychippus, 112; Mesohippus, 97, 112, 254; Orotherium, 253; Palæosyopous, 257; Palæotheriidæ, 251; Palæoplotherium, 254; Periptychus, 263; Phiolophus, 258-9; Protogonia, 263; Protohippus, 112, 254; Systemodon, 259-64. (See confusion in nomenclature, pp. 253-9.)
Horses, fossil, 95-93, 106-13; extinction of in South America, 107; recent discoveries of, 257-269; early progenitors of (Amblypoda) possibly carnivorous, 272.
Horses, "insane," 103.
Horses without ears, 103.
House, C. D., size of tooth-germs, 31; on teething, 47-8; grinders, 62; remnant teeth, 103, 104; removing a fractured tooth through the nostril, 103, 109; operations in Worcester, Mass., 109; idle talk about glanders, 19.; another probable mistake, 273
Hudson, E. D., Jr., mucous membrane, 213; ovaries, 213.
Hunter, J., theories of, 24-27; enamel of grinders, 63; attachment of teeth, 72; use of canines, 83; supernumerary teeth, 128; proving the formation of new dentine, 209.
Hughes, J., dimensions of teeth, 49; periosteum of teeth, 137.
Huxley, T. H., tapir, rhinoceros, and horse, 65-6; fossil horses, 110-11.
Hyohippus, fossil horse, 112.
Hyracotherium, fossil horse, 258-61.
Hyrax, teeth of and affinities with rhinoceros and elephant, 261.

Iguanodon, the, molars of, 63.
Incisors, the permanent, 53; length of, 57; curvatures of, 57; Chauveau's description of, 53-30; microscopic character of, 130-135.
Incisors, temporary, 47-52.
Inferior Maxillary Nerve, the, 223-24.

Jacobs, W., on elephant, 275.
Jaw, description of lower, 62.
Jaw Movements, changes in, 239.
Jaws, fractures of the, 94-213.
Jaws, human, chancres in, 99, 99-100.
Jennings, R., remnant tooth-germs and remnant teeth, 101.

Knowlson, J. C., bishoping, 211.
Koch, Robert, discovery of, 253.
Kölliker, Prof. Rudolf Albrecht, on tooth-germs, 39, 40, 46, 274.

Lafosse, Prof., dental cysts, 129.
Lambdotherium, fossil horse, 264-7.
Lampas, cause of, 88-91; lancing recommended for, 87, 91; burning for disapproved, 90-1.
Lancelet, the, comparison to, 81.
Lanzillotti Buonsanti, Prof., on dental cysts, 115-18.
Lecoq, Prof., canine follicles, 44; temporary canines, 52; description of grinders, 69-71; do. canines, 76-7; remnant teeth, 100.
Leeuwenhoek, discoveries of, 13.
Legros, C., experiments of, 27.
Leidy, J., letter from, 101; fossil teeth, 113; 257, 259; opinion of, 273.
Lincoln, A., 211.
Lion, the, canine teeth of, 83.
Liquor Sanguinis, the, 22, 242.
Lophiodon, teeth of, 258, 260.
Lubin, R., discovery of, 127.
Lyell, Mr., N. American fossil tooth corresponding to S. Amer., 110.

Macrops, Surg., experiences of, 117.
Madler, effect of on teeth, 24.
Magitot, E., 27; development of tooth-germs, human fœtus, 46.
Malpighi, discoveries of, 13.
Man, canine teeth of, 82, 83.
Man, early progenitors of, 80-3.
Manteodon, prophecy tooth of, 262.
Marks, dimensions of, 57. 53; twofold use of, 204; too much cement in, 209, 210.
Marsh, O. C., evolution of horse, 95-98; no 'mark' in teeth of early forms, 208; fossil birds' teeth, 114; description of mastodon and megatherium, 243; the Lophiodons, 253; Orohippus, 259.
Mastodon, the, 109, 114, 243.
May C., report of, 178, 179.
Mayhew, E, the cement, 17, 18; judging age by teeth, 207-8.
Mayo, Mr., experiments of, 218.
Megatherium, the, teeth of, 107, 108; description of, 243.
Melanian Races, teeth of, 99.
Membrana Nictitans, in early progenitors of man (Darwin), 82; nerve for in horse, 222; description of, 244.
Meniscotherium, fossil horse, 263-4.
Merychippus, fossil horse, 112.
Mesohippus, fossil horse, 97, 112.
Miocene period fossils of, 244.
Miohippus, fossil horse, 112.
Molars, bunodont, 203.
Molars, selenodont, 263.
Molars, the, 54; inclination of, 54; description of, 69-71; microscopical character of, 130-35.
Moon-Blindness, cause of, 105.

## INDEX.

Moore, T., a mountain herb, 25.
Morphology, definition of, 245.
Morton, Prof., treatise by, 193.
Mules' Teeth, telling age by, 215.
Müller, Prof., discovery of, 14-5.
Muntjac-Deer, 78, 246.
Musk-Deer, 78, 245.
Mylodon, the, 108, 246.

NARWHAL, the, tushes of, 79; description of, 246.
Nature barricading disease, 139, 209.
Newberry, J. S., zoology, 256.
Niebuhr, opinion of, 25.
Nippers, the, use of word, 47.
Nomenclature, confusion in, 258-9.

ODONTOBLASTS, the, 31.
Odontolithos, the, 17, 247.
Odontornithes (birds), teeth of, 114.
Odontonecrosis, 138.
Odontrypy, operation of, 139.
Ohlinger, O. P., discovery of, 113.
Ophthalmic Nerve, the, 219-22.
Ornithorhynchus, the, 80, 247.
Operating, rules for, 154-160.
Oreste, Surg., discovery of, 178.
Orohippus, fossil horse, teeth of, 96, large tushes of, 97; toes of, 97; size of animal, 112; name of, 259.
Osteo-sarcoma, case of, 186.
Owen, R., dental science, 8, 10, 12-22; tooth-germs, 32-37; breadth and thickness, 49; temporary canines, 51; teething, 55; description of grinders, 64-68; teeth of anoplothere, 65; do. ruminants, 65; do. tapir, 65; do. rhinoceros, 6 ; do. megatherium, 107; remnant teeth, 102; fossil horses' teeth, 103-104; microscopical appearance of horses' teeth, 130-135; diseases of teeth, 137; diseased fossil tooth, 173, 174; the fifth pair of nerves, 223, 224; discovers Hyracotherium, 258; teeth of elephant, 275; tooth-vascularity, 29; probable circulation and prolongation of nerves in dentinal tubes, 30.

PALEONTOLOGY, definition of, 248.
Paleosyopous, fossil horse, 267.
Paleothere, teeth of, 68.
Paleotheriidæ, fossil horses, 261.
Parker, Willard, on caries, 221.
Parnell, C., remnant teeth, 102.
Parrot-Mouth, 157, 168.
Pathology of the Teeth, 133-174.
Percival, W., teething, 80-83; lampas, 83-92; diseases of teeth, 133, 135; ophthalmic ganglion, 221.
Periosteum, elasticity of, 73, 74; definition of, 249-50.
Periptychus, a fossil horse with teeth resembling a serpent's, 263.

Perissodactyla (odd-toed mammals), 237-64.
Pessina, Prof., discovery of, 215.
Phenacodus (earliest fossil horse), description of, 260-264.
Pierce, Dr., opinion of, 287.
Plasse, M., mouth-screw 156.
Pliocene (period), fossils of, 250.
Pliohippus, fossil horse, size of, 112; confusion in name of, 259.
Pliolophus, fossil horse, 258-9.
Pony, great suffering of a, 201.
Portal, learning of, 14.
Pouchet, M., tooth-germs, 274.
Premolar, reasons for use of word, 53; inclination of the, 54.
Processes, alveolar, diseases of, 166.
Protogonia, fossil horse, 263.
Protohippus, fossil horse, 112, 264.
Public Opinion, 287-92.
Pulp, the tooth, 31.
Pulpal Cavity, relation of, 22.
Purkinji, discoveries of, 14, 16; corpuscles of, 9; cells of, 16.

QUADRUMANA, the, 86, 81, 251.
Quain, Jonas, fifth nerve and ophthalmic ganglion, 220.

RAMSEY, J., skill of, 104.
Raoux, C., obligation to, 28.
Rénault, Robt., report of, 187-92.
Regimen, 162-164.
Retzius, Prof., discoveries and conjectures of, 16, 19, 20, 21.
Revel, M., report of, 197.
Reversion, doctrine of, 80.
Rhinoceros, the, teeth of, 67.
Rhinoceros, the woolly, 251.
Rich, Dr., children's teeth, 277.
Riders, first nations of, 273.
Rigot, temporary canines, 52.
Robin, C., dog tooth-germs, 27.
Rockwell, E. A., report of, 277.
Roder, Surgeon, on dental cysts, 118.
Roudanoosky, M., on nerves, 218.
Rousseau, M., cutting milk teeth, 48.
Ruminants, teeth of, 65; four stomachs of, 252.
Ruini, discovery of, 69.
Ryder, J. A., treatise of, 268.

SANTY, A. H., report of, 180.
Satterthwaite, T. E., on corpuscles, 233-4; on tubercles, 255.
Scelidothere, remains of, 109.
Schaaffhausen, shortened jaws, 99.
Schwann, Dr., researches of, 20.
Seelye Prof., correlation forces, 234.
Selection, natural, 98.
Selection, sexual, 98.
Sewell, W., dental cysts, 122.
Shark, fossil, teeth of, 236.
Simonds, Prof., lever-forceps, 156.
Sinuses, valves, osseous plates, &c.,

of, 152; gutta-percha as a filling for, 177.
Smith, W., report of, 182-184.
Speculum Oris, use of, 149.
Spencer H., evolution, 237.
Star, dentinal, 59, 209.
Stone, case of in horse's jaw, 193.
Strong, Dr., translation by, 274.
Superior Maxillary Nerve, the, 222.
Supernumerary Teeth, 127-129; 139.
Surmon, H., report of, 177.
Swallowing a Diseased Tooth, death of a horse from, 187 192.
Swallowing a heathy tooth, 193.
Systemodon, fossil horse, 259, 260-4.

TABLES OF GRINDERS, the, 61.
Teeth, abnormal, cases of beneath right kidney and near right ear of a lamb, 116-17; on mastoid process of temporal bone, posterior part of sphenoid bone and in testicle, 117; in ovaries, orbit, palate, tongue, side of jaw, cheek and neck, 119; base of ear, 124.
Teeth, absorption roots of, 48, 70-1, 275-6, 238.
Teeth, canine (horses'), description and probable extinction of, 75-77.
Teeth, canine, use of in different animals, 77-85; made to tear flesh, 271.
Teeth, constant in the same type, and generally appreciably modified according to family, 12.
Teeth, continuous growth of, 73, 143; extraction on account of, 178.
Teeth, deciduous, retention of, 129.
Teeth, elephant, unique mode of cutting and shedding several dentitions, 274-6 ; size, structure, &c., 274-6; great quantity cement in, 10.
Teeth, elephant (Indian), indications of age by, 275.
Teeth emanating from osseous system, 121.
Teeth, foals', absorption of roots of, non-continuous growth of, scarcity of cement on crowns of, 48; crowns worn off by attrition rather than shed, 50; breadth of, 49.
Teeth, fossil birds', 114.
Teeth, fossil elephant, weight of, 276.
Teeth, fossil horses' (see "Horses, fossil." p. 281).
Teeth, fossil horses' (South and N. American), 10 -19.
Teeth, goats', gold and silver hues produced in, 25-6.
Teeth, growing, effect of madder on, white red and white, 25.
Teeth, horses', anomalous condition of, 142.
Teeth, horses', dimensions of, 71.

Teeth, horses', discovery that they indicate age, 215.
Teeth, horses', fillings for, 164.
Teeth, horses', signs of improvement in, 266, 271.
Teeth, horses' (Spanish), peculiarities of, 215.
Teeth, horses', temporary, 47-52; permanent, 53-74; canines, 75-88; remnant, 94-114; abnormal, 115-127; supernumerary, 139; under the microscope, 180-185; pathology of, 136-174; dentistry of, 175-193; indicators of age, 108-215.
Teeth, human, changes in, 99.
Teeth, in harmony with general system, 11.
Teeth, mules', telling age by (differing somewhat from horse), 215.
Teeth, readily preserved in a fossil state, 12.
Teeth, remnant, 94; regarded as phenomenons, 94, 101; line of descent, 94; not to be confounded with supernumeraty teeth, 94; the name, 94; easily lost, 99-100.
Teeth, rudimentary, 99; why good teachers, 99.
Teeth, supernumerary, 127-8, 139.
Teeth, three sets of, 128.
Teeth, transplanting of, 26-29.
Teeth, tubes (hollow columns) of, 12.
Teeth, value of to the anatomist, 11.
Teeth, variety and use of, 10, 11.
Teeth, various animals', Boar, 77, 84; Cachalot, 79; Camel, 66, 78; Cattle, 91-2; Chevrotain, 78, 232; Coluber Scaber, 121; Copybara (or Capybara), 10, 233; Dinoceras mirabilis (fossil) 236; Dugong, 79, 235; Elephant, 77, 274; do, fossil, 244; Hippopotamus, 63; Hog, 63; Hyrax, 260; Iguanodon, 63; Lion, 83; Mastodon, 109, 243; Megatherium, 107, 243; Muntjac deer, 78, 245; Musk-deer, 78, 245; Narwhal, 79, 246; Ornithorhynchus, 80, 247; Rhinoceros, 67; Ruminants, 65, 252; Shark (fossil), 226; Tapir, 65; Toxodon, 109, 254; Walrus, 77; Zebra, 52.
Teeth, vascularity of, 22-30; nerves and circulating vessels of, 26.
Teeth, wolf, why called remnant, 94.
Tenon, verifies Ruini's discovery, 69.
Tennyson's "gulf of doubt," 270.
Toes, 97, 112, 265; cause of reduction in number, 269; form a semicircle when applied to the ground, 269.
Tomes, C. S., tooth-germs, 37-41; temporary canines, 52; dentine, enamel, and cement, 63; attachment of teeth, 73; tushes of bears, 84-5, evolution, 98-9; no 'mark' in teeth of early fossil horses, 203.

## INDEX. 285

Tomes, J., a tooth barricading disease, 189.
Tooth, abnormal, description of, 123.
Tooth, a diseased fossil, 173-4.
Tooth, a fractured, 193-9.
Tooth, a prophecy, 202.
Tooth, a whale's, description of, 79.
Tooth, elephant, in Worth's Museum (New York), 275.
Tooth in upper jaw of a bull, 127.
Tooth, nature of, 7, 8; iridescence of, 12, 16; no inherent power of reparation in, 137.
Tooth Pulp, description of, 81
Tooth, remnant, vicious inclination of a, 104.
Tooth, swallowing a diseased (fatal), 187-192.
Tooth, swallowing a healthy, 193.
Tooth-Cough, treatment for, 92.
Tooth-Germs, development of, 31-46.
Tooth-Germs, cogs'. grafting whole germs, separate enamel organs, dentine caps, &c., in dogs and guinea-pigs, those in the latter animal failing, 27-8.
Tooth-Germs, elephant, 274.
Tooth Germs, human, transformations of epithelial and enamel germs, dentine bulbs, caps, &c., in, from 7th to 39th week, 46.
Tooth-Tumor, unusual case of, 196.
Tooth and Bone, analogy of, 23.
Toxodon, remains of, 109; description of, 254.
Trephine, the, 254.
Trephining Sinuses, 157-161.
Trigeminus Nerve (in the horse), description of, 216-226.
Tripier, M., resection of nerves, 217.
Trocar, the, 255.
Tushes, fighting with, in various animals, 77-85.
Tushes horses', practically useless, 75; different from other teeth, 75; distances from incisors and grinders, 75, 75; shape and dimensions of, 76; curvature of roots, 76.
Tushes, removal of, 155.
Tushes, size of in Orohippus, 97.
Tusks, elephant fighting with, 77; varying curvatures, weight, length, &c., of, 276.
Tuttle, R. M., on evolution, 270-2.

VARNELL, G., opinion of, 102; diseases of teeth, 138. 136; the sinuses, 152, 153, 161 ; caries, 164-166; diseases of alveolar processes, 166; parrot-mouth, 167; osteo-sarcoma, 186-7; fractured jaws, 194.
Views of an evolutionist, 270-2.

WALLACE, A. R., cause of destruction of ungulata, 111; fossil horses, 112; geology, 240.
Walrus, the, mode of fighting of, 77.
Walsh, J. H., age by teeth, 208.
Wedges, scientific, use of, 271.
West, bone-beds of the, 257.
Wheeler, Capt., report on survey of, 261-2.
Williams, Prof. W., teething, 91; remnant teeth, 104, 105; dental cysts, 125-127; caries, 169-171.
Williams, W., necrosis, 246.
Winter, J. H., use of tushes, 85.
Wolf-teeth, why a good generic name, 94.
Woodward, J. J., tooth pulp, 81; histology, 241.
Woolly Rhinoceros, (fossil), 251.
Works, general, 4.
Works, special, 4, 290.
Wortman, J. L., on fossil horses, 257-269; discovery of, 260.
Wyman, Prof. discovery of, 81.

YATES, L. G., fossil elephant teeth, 276.
Youatt, W., sugar as food, 30; tooth-germs, 44, 45; infundibula of grinders. 58; description of lower jaw, 62 ; use of tushes, 84; teething, 85, 86; lampas, 90, 91; cropping horses' ears. 103; remnant teeth, 105; food, 102-104 ; diseases of teeth, 172, 173; fractured jaws, 196-198; 'mark' of central nippers, 205; difficulties of judging age, 207; bishoping, 210; trud' tricks, 212, 214; crib-biting, 212, 213; indications of age independent of teeth, 214; fifth pair of nerves, 216-225; cæcum, 230; colon, 232; membrana nictitans, 244; solipeds. 253.
Youmans, E. L., evolution, 237.

ZEBRA, temporary canine teeth of, 52.
Zoölogy, definition of, 256.

# PUBLIC OPINION.

HORSES' TEETH.—Such is the title of a work we have just read with considerable interest, because it embraces much that is instructive and useful. Designed as the publication is to give a synopsis of the fundamental principles of dental science, it has a defect attributable to the author's lack of practical experience in the specialty of which he treats. * * * The chapter on canine teeth contains much of interest, and fully sustains the theory that horses suffer from febrile irritations, as the result of interrupted dentition, and that the free use of the lance is as serviceable as when used on an obstructed eye-tooth of a child. The disease known as lampas, which is often accompained by a distressing cough, and which so seriously interferes with feeding, is shown to be due to the same cause and to require the same remedy. To state that caries most frequently proceeds from inflammation beginning in the pulp-cavity, or that caries of the roots is the result of inflammation of the alveolo-dental periosteum, is certainly far from the experience of the practical dentist; but, notwithstanding these defects, there is much of value in this (the eighth chapter) as well as the succeeding chapters on the dentistry of the teeth, their indications of age, their nerves, &c. * * *.—*C. N. Pierce in "Dental Cosmos."*

"HORSES' TEETH," by Wm. H. Clarke of New York, is a neat and handsomely bound volume, containing selections from the very best authors, with appropriate additions by the author, making a book that is invaluable to veterinary surgeons, and of great practical benefit to dentists, and should be studied by every person who treats the teeth. The author treats of the teeth from the time of the formation of the germ to their full development, and gives their pathology and dentistry also. A vocabulary of the technical terms used forms a valuable addition.—*Dental News.*

This work is undoubtedly in advance of anything heretofore published on the subject in this country. * * * When the author says that "probably the temporary teeth are absorbed by the permanent," he displays the folly of attempting to write on a subject that one does not understand.* Still the work is useful and will probably aid in the elevation of veterinary surgery.—*Missouri Dental Journal.*

This book is in a great measure a compilation from works on dentistry, anatomy, physiology, microscopy and veterinary surgery, as they relate to the development, structure and care of the teeth of horses. As we are a believer in horse dentistry, we have looked over the work with much pleasure and no inconsiderable profit.—*Dental Advertiser.*

This book is a venture in the field of veterinary science which we hope to see more frequently imitated. It is mainly a compilation, admirably arranged, and prepared with great thoroughness of detail. The compiled matter is well selected and condensed, much of it being rewritten. It contains much besides the matter pertaining to horses' teeth, the teeth of many other animals being described and compared with those of the horse; in fact, the work might be entitled "Teeth" instead of "Horses' Teeth." It gives a history of the evolution of the horse from early geological periods, the wolf-teeth, which the author has named "Remnant Teeth," being traced back to the Eocene period, when they were functionally developed. This fact throws light on what has been a mystery, and the author appears to have made a discovery.

The work, as a whole, is very commendable, and we feel

---

* See pages 48 and 50. A few changes have been made and some fresh matter added. But I will venture to ask the editor of the *Journal* what becomes of the *roots* of a temporary tooth when the shell of its *crown* when shed is sometimes not more than the sixteenth of an inch in thickness? What becomes of the roots of elephant teeth? (See pages 274-5-6.)

sure it will find a place in the library of all interested in a thoroughly practical as well as scientific knowledge of horses' teeth, and will be found especially valuable both to the student and practitioner of comparative medicine and surgery.—*Journal of Comparative Medicine and Surgery.*

The work consists mainly of quotations from standard writers. It is very interesting and instructive reading, and is fully worth the small sum it costs. The author deserves credit for his labor in collecting information from so many separate sources, and presenting it in so small a compass and so readable a form. However, there are errors in the vocabulary that ought to be corrected.—*Veterinary Gazette.*

It possesses the merit of presenting in a condensed form, for the study of the veterinary surgeon, the anatomy, pathology, and reparative surgery of horses' teeth, and to him it will save much labor and furnish a ready reference, and hence be an efficient aid. * * *—*Medical Gazette.*

* * * The work contains an immense amount of useful information, and as it fills an unoccupied field, ought to be successful.—*Medical Record.*

We understand this book is having a rapid sale among horsemen. Hereafter we suppose the title H. D. D. will become common. How nicely Mr. Clarke tells us of the cutting and shedding of the temporary and permanent dentitions. In the future we expect that greater attention will be given to the teeth.—*North American Journal of Homeopathy.*

Horses' Teeth.—Owners of all classes of horses should be in possession of a remarkably useful work entitled "Horses' Teeth," by Wm. H. Clarke. The work is based on the best authorities on odontology and veterinary science, and arranged in an easy, comprehensive form. With a view of rendering technical terms readily understood, a vocabulary of the medical and technical terms is attached. Dental science, as hitherto expounded, has never afforded horse owners the instruction it professes to aim at. The trouble has been the use of technical phrases. Mr. Clarke, alive to the necessity of giving to the public a popular treatise, has presented a work which must find its way in all circles, and, above all, reach the understanding of the average reader.—*Turf, Field and Farm.*

THIS work deals with horses' teeth in a very complete manner, and will doubtless be found of great value by students of veterinary science. It is a compilation, but Mr. Clarke has done his work in a careful manner. * * * A study of this work cannot fail to be of value to all who are interested in the horse.—*London (Eng.) Live Stock Journal.*

THE book is compiled from the best authorities.—*Rural New Yorker.*

HORSES' TEETH.—We have received from Mr. W. H. Clarke a duodecimo volume containing a compilation of everything valuable that has been written by the best known odontologists. * * * The so-called "wolf-teeth" are traced to the horse which existed previous to the pliocene period. Mr. Clarke calls them "remnant" teeth. * * * The work is a valuable addition to veterinary science.—*The Country Gentleman.*

IT is a venture in the field of veterinary science, and, though in general a compilation, will be found of great practical service, and in its present form a new thing. It will be of use especially to horsemen and farmers.—*Massachusetts Ploughman.*

THIS work is mainly compiled, but the selections evince care, judgment, research, and discrimination. It will prove valuable to the veterinary student and practitioner.—*Pen and Plow.*

HAD this work been issued prior to Huxley's "Crayfish" or Comte's "Sight" it would have been deemed too special. The subject is scientifically treated, with a decided tendency toward the practical. * * *.—*Syracuse Standard.*

HORSES' TEETH.—* * * Mr. Clarke devotes considerable space to descriptions of the different classes of teeth. * * * Although there is a great deal of technical language in the work the copious vocabulary at its close renders it practical for those who wish to learn about the structure and diseases of the teeth, and the method of treating them under various circumstances. Many instances are quoted from good authorities in which horses have been treated for diseases of the jaw, and the methods by means of which they were cured are carefully set forth. We present some extracts from the chapter on the teeth as indicators of age. (See pp. 204-5.) The treatment of this subject is only an example of the fullness and accuracy of the entire work.— *Utica Herald.*

Mr. W. H. Clarke's "Horses' Teeth" is a complete and interesting treatise which may be accepted at once as both a useful manual of equine dentistry and an agreeable study of certain aspects of comparative zoology. Every possible deformity or peculiarity observable in the teeth of the horse, as well as every roguery practiced on them by dishonest dealers is fully handled, and a succinct account is given of all the maladies of the teeth themselves, and of other organs with which the teeth have a functional relation.—*New York Herald.*

The treatise on horses' teeth by William H. Clarke, a metropolitan journalist, has already attracted wide attention, and is an invaluable work in its way. Great care and much labor have been bestowed in its preparation, and the book supplies a want that has long been felt by horsemen, farmers and the student and practitioner of comparative medicine and surgery. —*New York Graphic.*

The title so fully describes the scope of the volume that little need be added except criticism. The author is frank enough to admit professional inexperience, but has made the topic of the work a matter of careful investigation for a year. He has wisely deferred to the opinions of naturalists and veterinary surgeons, and quotes liberally from their works in every chapter, thus supplying a cyclopedic stock of information bearing directly on horses' teeth in health and disease, which is very convenient for those who keep or raise horses, and the average veterinary surgeon.—*Phrenological Journal.*

The thoroughness of detail with which every point relating to the subject of this work is treated will impress every one with its reliability and value. It is undoubtedly true that much suffering, disease and death have resulted from ignorance of what is herein given, and that much unintentional cruelty to horses may be prevented by studying this volume.

Though the title implies that the work is confined exclusively to the teeth of horses, it is not so; the teeth of other animals claim nearly as much attention as those of the horse. The theory of evolution is introduced, the history of the horse being traced from the Eocene period, when the wolf or "remnant" teeth were functionally developed. The book will be prized by all who seek the welfare and happiness not only of the human race, but of all sentient beings.—*Banner of Light.*

WE all know that horses suffer with their teeth, and the work gives full instructions as to their care. * * * The author is an evolutionist, and has devoted much study to fossil horses.—*New Orleans Times.*

PRACTICAL BOOKS.—" Horses' Teeth," is a valuable treatise that ought to be in the possession of horsemen, farmers, and veterinarians. * * *.—*Pittsburg Commercial Gazette.*

DR. C. F. HOEING (Jersey City Hights, N. J.) says: "After a careful reading of your book, 'Horses' Teeth,' I wish to say that it appears to me to be an able compilation of scientific facts, and a basis for further investigation of horse dentistry by the profession; at the same time containing valuable information for intelligent horsemen and farmers, as well as naturalists generally. I miss only very valuable information to be found in numerous German books."

DR. J. M. HEARD, 205 Lexington Ave., New York, says: "The book is full of valuable information; in fact, one would search a single library in vain to obtain it. None but those who have performed similar work can appreciate the immense amount of labor expended in its preparation. No student or practitioner can afford to be without it."

Dr. B S. Brewster of Norwich, Conn., says: "I have been an advocate of horse dentistry for thirty years, even arguing against veterinary surgeons. Thank God, light has come at last."

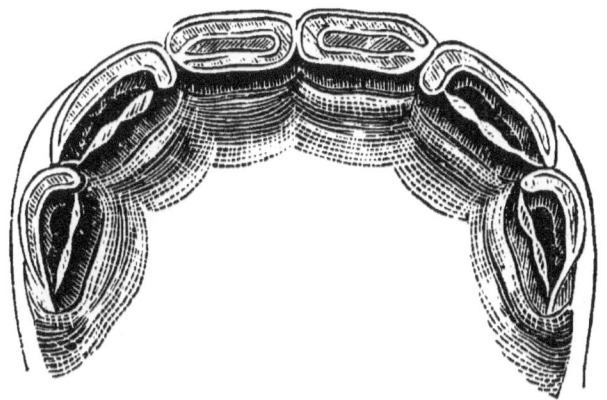

1-Year-Old, Lower Jaw (*Brandt*).

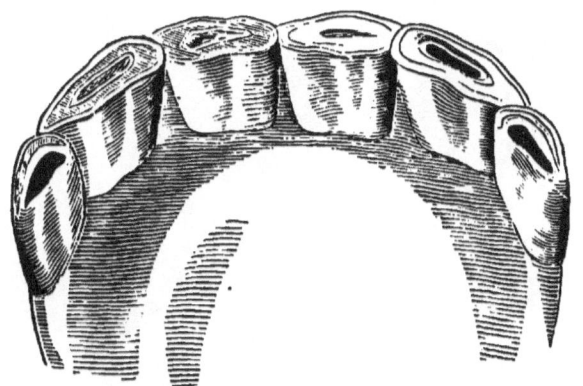

2-Year-Old, Lower Jaw; drawn from Nature.

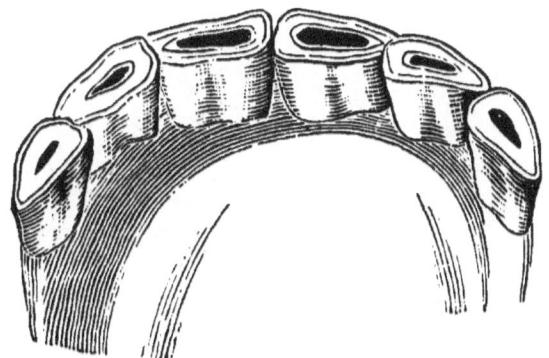

3-Year-Old, Lower Jaw; drawn from Nature.

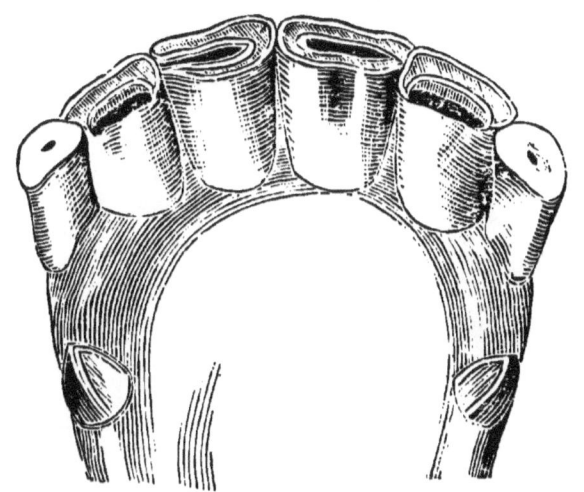

4-Year-Old, Lower Jaw; drawn from Nature.

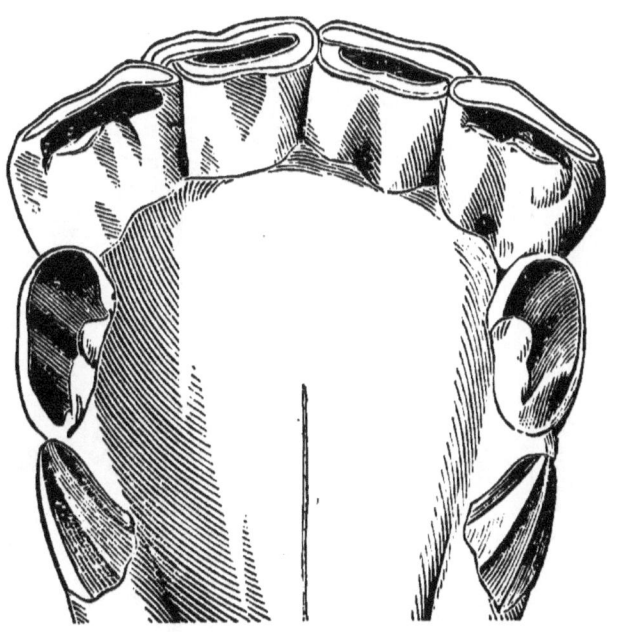

5-Year-Old, Lower Jaw; drawn from Nature.

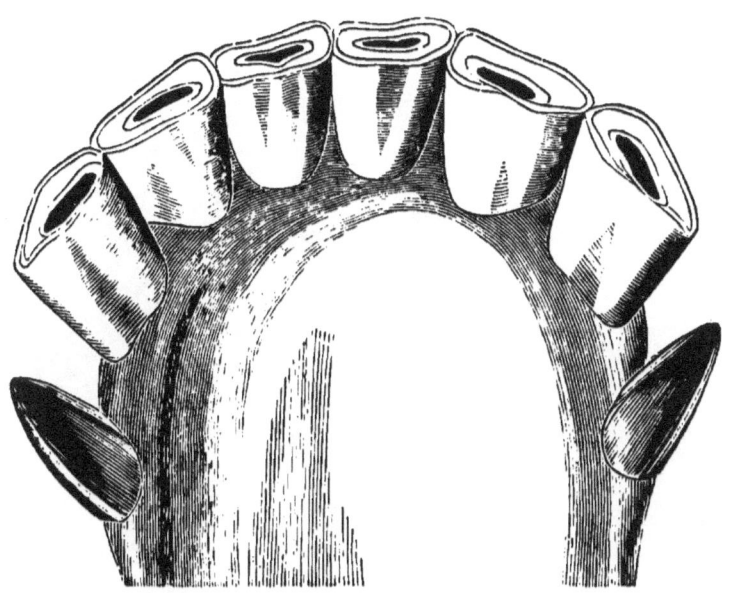

6-Year-Old, Lower Jaw; drawn from Nature.

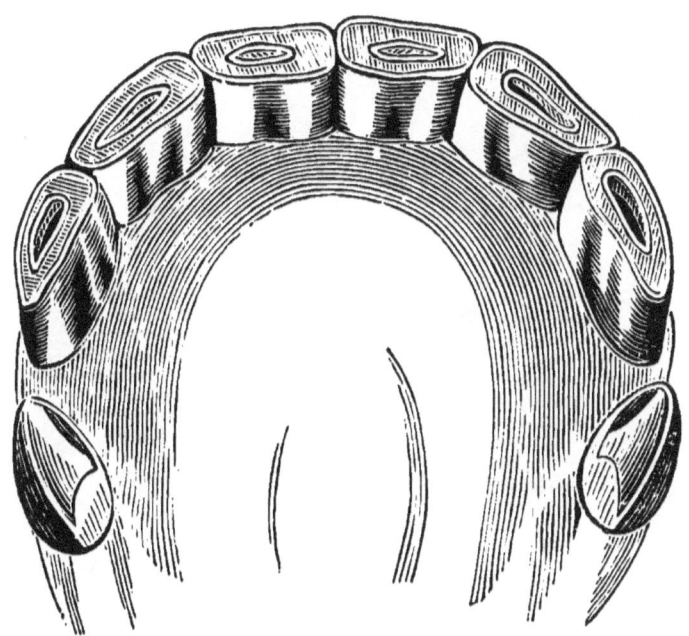

7-Year-Old. Lower Jaw (*Brandt*).

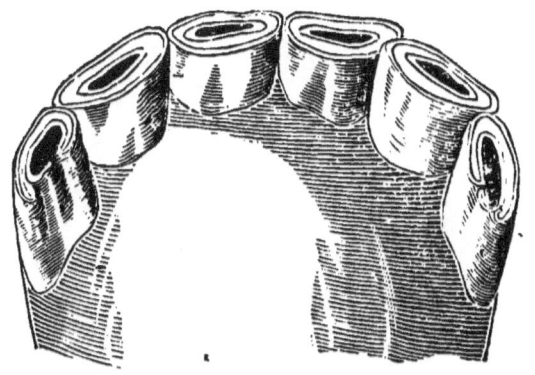

8-Year-Old, Upper Jaw (*Walsh*). About ⅔ nat. size.

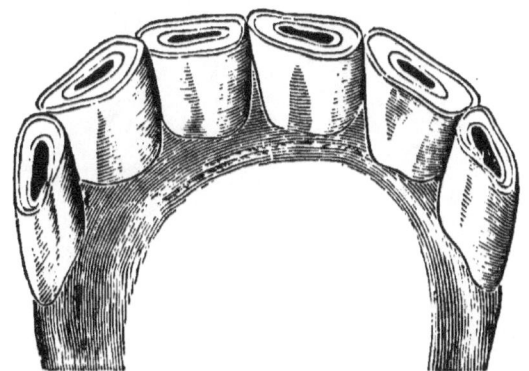

9-Year-Old, Upper Jaw (*Walsh*). About ⅔ nat. size.

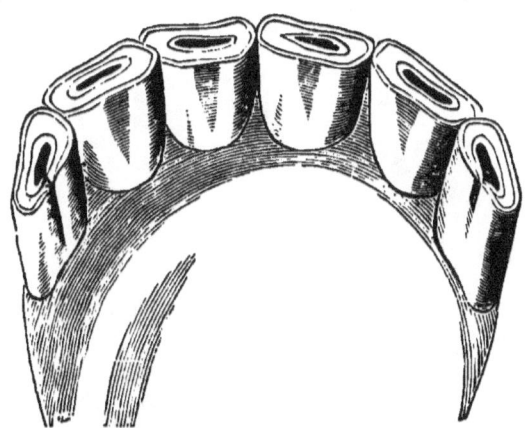

10-Year-Old, Upper Jaw (*Walsh*). About ⅔ nat. size.

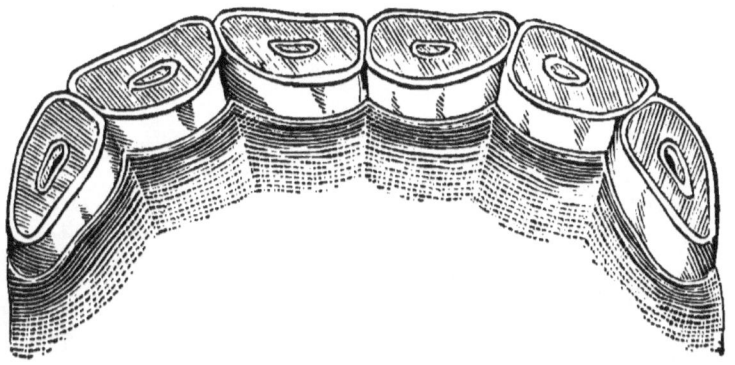

11 years, Upper Jaw. The marks have disappeared.

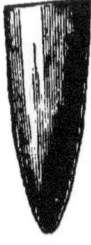

The Mark, dissected as it were. (See page 58.)

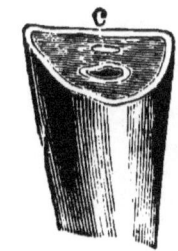

*c*, The Dentinal star, sometimes mistaken for the mark. (See page 209.)

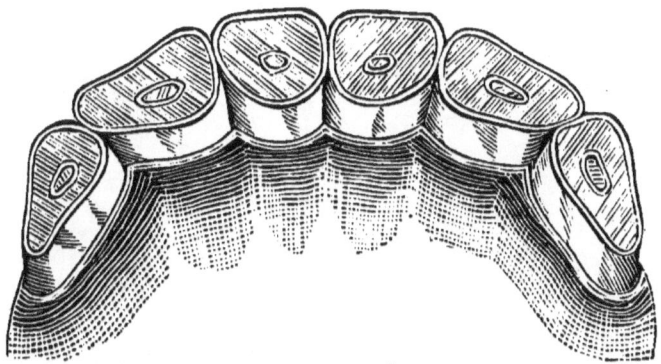

12 years, Lower Jaw. Change in shape is now clearly defined. The respective pairs (centrals, dividers, corners) assume in turn (from 12 years till old age) various shapes—semi-square, rounded, triangular, wedge-shaped, etc.

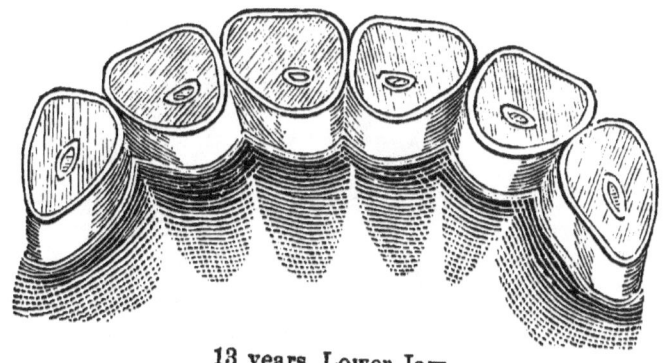

13 years, Lower Jaw.

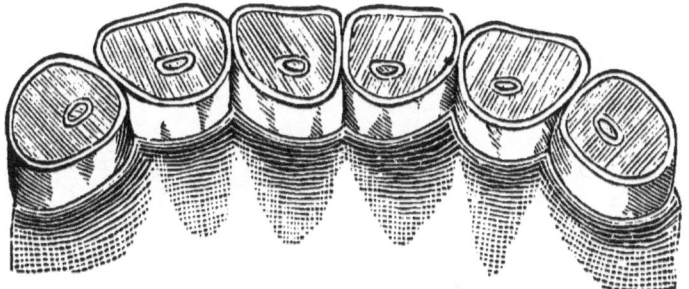

14 years, Lower Jaw.

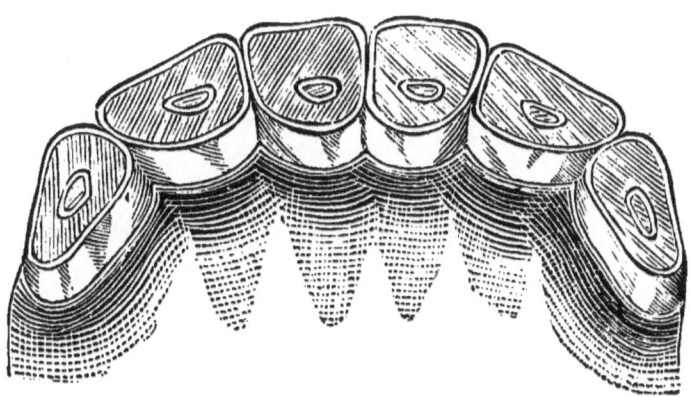

15 years, Upper Jaw.

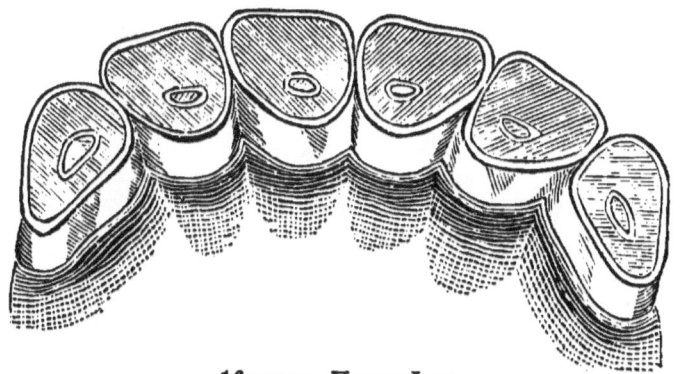

16 years, Upper Jaw.

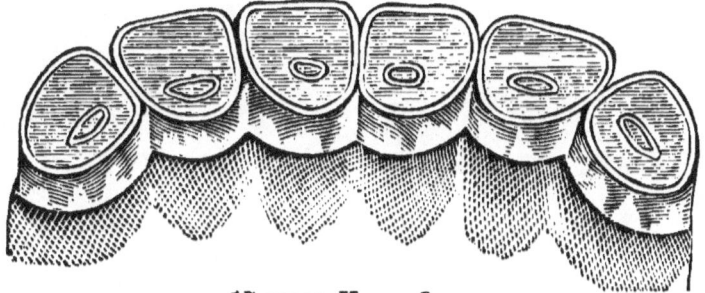

17 years, Upper Jaw.

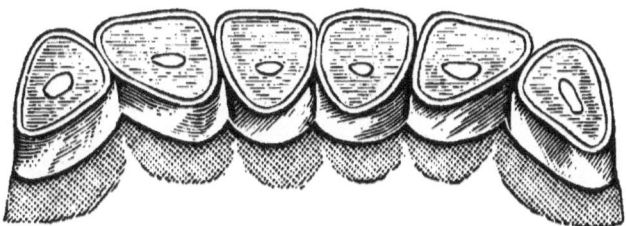

18 years, Lower Jaw.

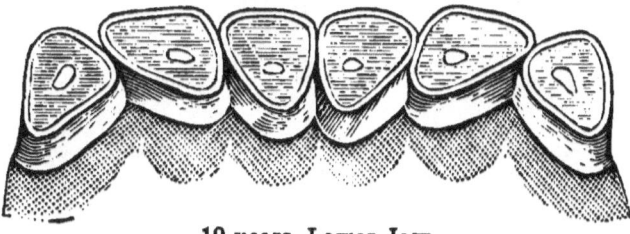

19 years, Lower Jaw.

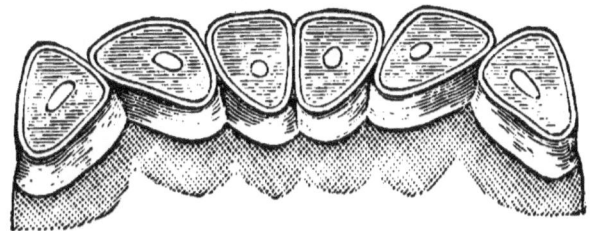

20 years, Lower Jaw.

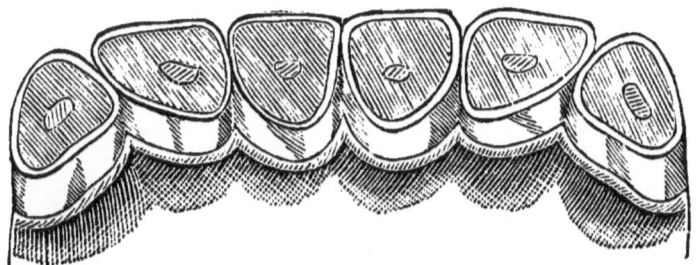

21 years, Upper Jaw.

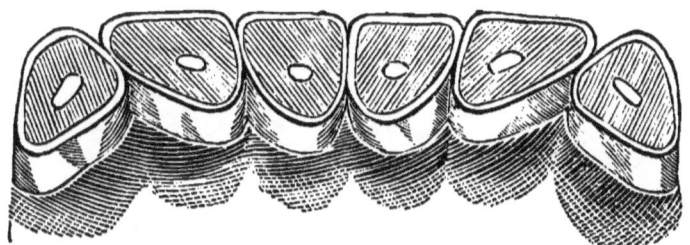

22 years, Upper Jaw.

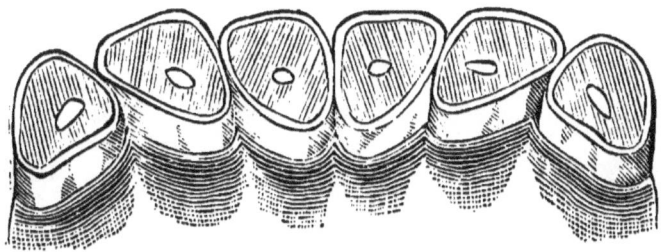

28 years, Upper Jaw.

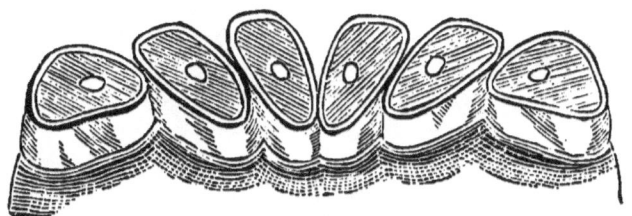

24 years, Lower Jaw.

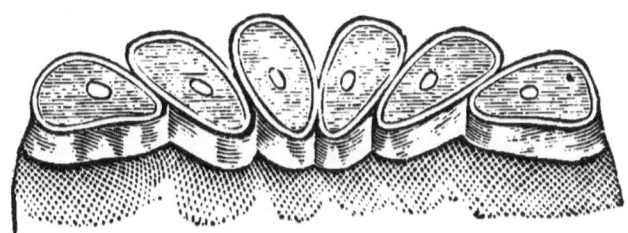

25 years, Lower Jaw.

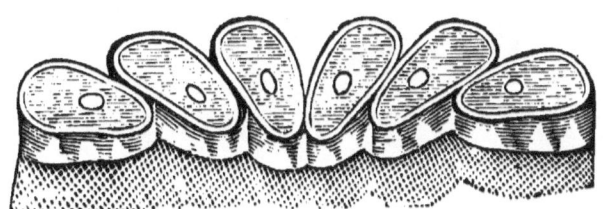

26 years, Lower Jaw.

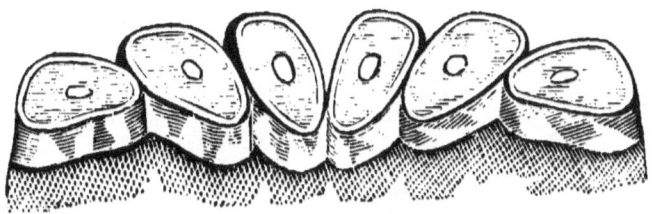

27 years, Upper Jaw.

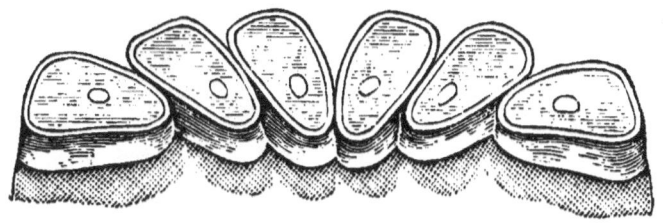

28 years, Upper Jaw.

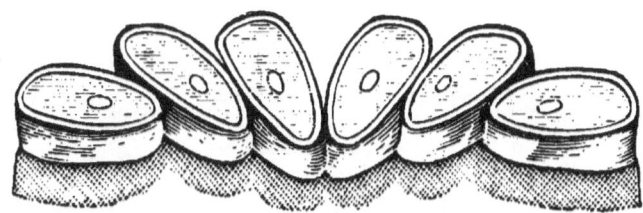

29 years, Upper Jaw.

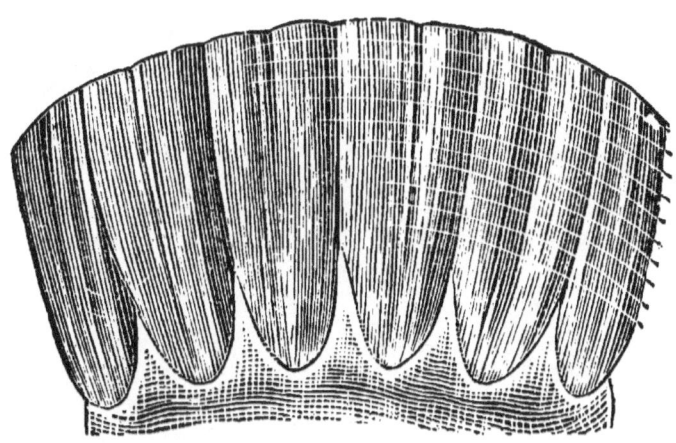

A Parrot-Mouth (lower jaw). The ten lines represent ten years' growth. The marks, having never been worn, represent a 6-year-old. The horse is therefore 16 years old. (This cut, as well as many of the preceding, is from Brandt's "Age of Horses.")

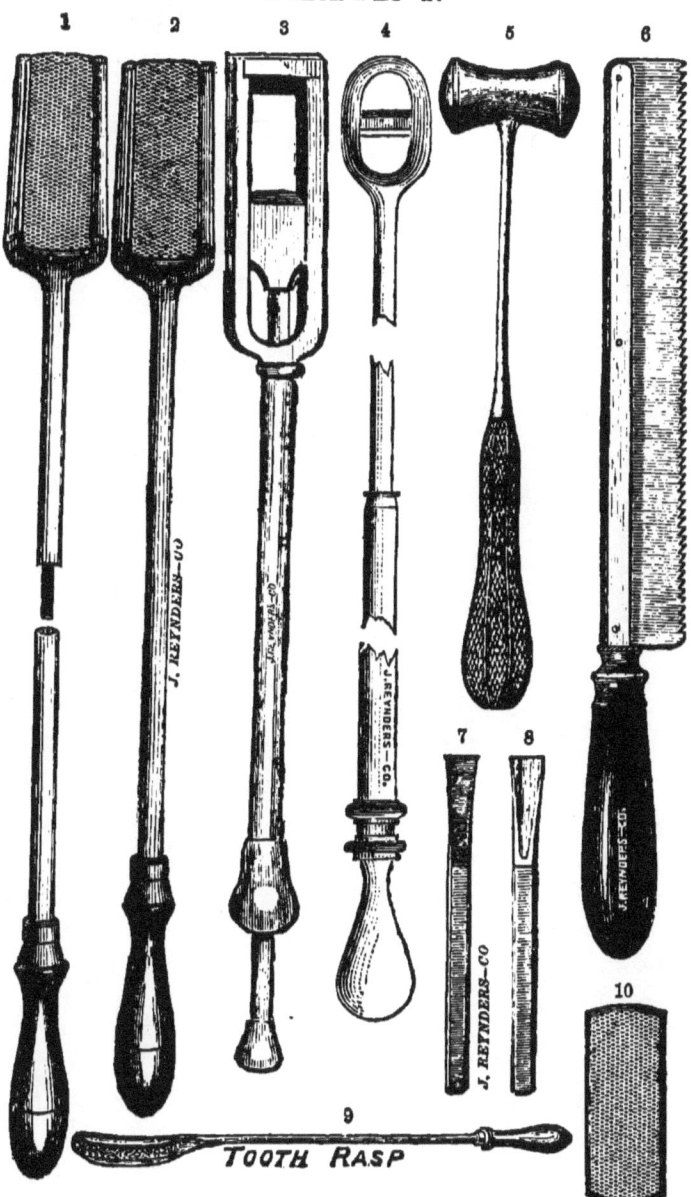

## PLATE II.

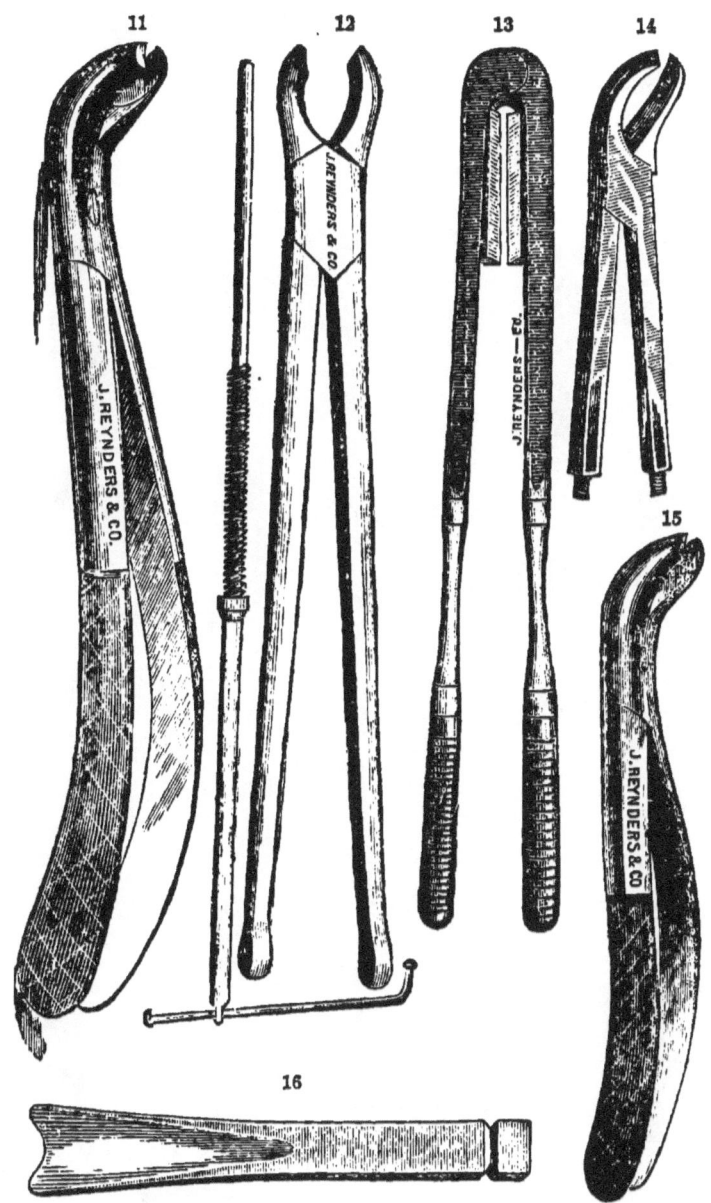

PLATE III.

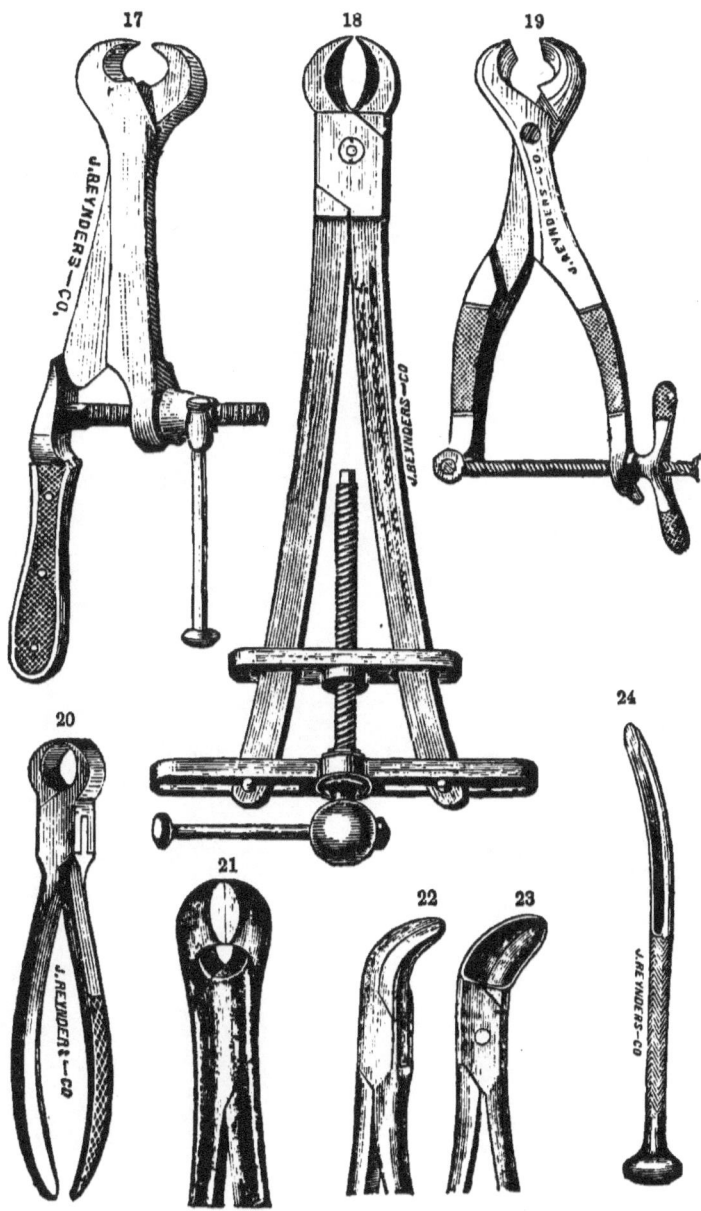

# PLATE IV.

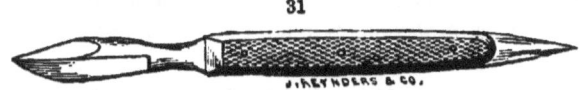

# John Reynders & Co.,

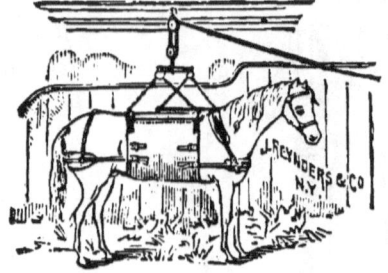

## MANUFACTURERS AND IMPORTERS OF

# Veterinary Instruments

### OF SUPERIOR QUALITY AND WORKMANSHIP.

## Slings for Suspending Animals

### A SPECIALTY.

## No. 303 Fourth Avenue,

### New York.

---

## Price List of Veterinary Dental Instruments Illustrated in this book.

| | | | |
|---|---|---|---|
| Plate I. | Fig. 1. Adjustable Tooth File; in handle to unscrew, | $4.00 |
| " | " 2. " " " in stiff handle......  | 3.00 |
| | House's " " in handle to unscrew, | 4.00* |
| | House's " " in stiff handle........ | 3.00* |
| " | " 3. Prof. Going's Tooth Chisel .................. | 17.50 |
| " | " 4. French Model " " .................. | 14.00 |
| " | " 5. Tooth Mallet, lead filled, not rebounding...... | 2.50 |
| " | " 6. French Model Tooth Saw ...................... | 3.50 |
| " | " 7. Narrow Tooth Chisel, length 5 inches ......... | 1.25 |

| | | | |
|---|---|---|---|
| *Plate I.* | Fig. 8. Narrow Tooth Gouge, length 5 inches ......... | $1.50 |
| " | " 9. Tooth Rasp guarded; in stiff handle........... | 3.00* |
| | " " " in handle to unscrew.... | 3.75* |
| | " " plain; in stiff handle ............ | 1.75* |
| | " " plain; in handle to unscrew....... | 2.50* |
| " | " 10. Extra Blade for Adjustable Tooth File.......... | 0.40 |
| | Extra Blade for House's " " .......... | 0.40* |
| *Plate II.* | " 11. Heavy Tooth Forceps, length 15 inches........ | 5.50 |
| " | " 12. Prof. Going's Tooth Forceps with closing screw and crank handle........................ | 25.00 |
| " | " 13. House's Tooth Cutting Forceps, | |
| " | " 14. House's Tooth Pulling Forceps, one set of removable handles to both | } 28.00 |
| " | " 15. Wolf Tooth Forceps, length 9 inches........... | 3.50 |
| " | " 16. Wide Tooth Chisel, length 10 inches........... | 2.00 |
| | " " " " 16 " ............ | 3.00 |
| *Plate III.* | " 17. Tooth Cutting Forceps, French model ........ | 25.00 |
| " | " 18. " " " Möller's ............... | 32.00 |
| " | " 19. " " " French model ......... | 20.50 |
| " | " 20. House's Tooth Cutting Forceps............... | 6.50 |
| " | " 21. " " " " ............... | 6.50 |
| " | " 22. " " " " ............... | 6.50 |
| " | " 23. " " " " ............... | 6.50 |
| " | " 24. Narrow Tooth Gouge, with steel head.......... | 2.00 |
| *Plate IV.* | " 25. Bow Tooth Saw, with two blades.............. | 6.00 |
| " | " 26. Tooth Key, with hooks of assorted sizes ....... | 35.00 |
| " | " 27. Plain Tooth Saw............................. | 1.50 |
| " | " 28. Chain Tooth Saw ............................ | 12.50 |
| " | " 29. Fine ferruled Tooth Saw...................... | 1.75 |
| " | " 30. Narrow Tooth Chisel, length 6 inches .......... | 1.25 |
| " | " 31. Hurlburt's Gum Knife and Tooth Pick ........ | 2.00 |

**Our Alphabetical Register of Veterinary Instruments of 90 Pages and containing about 325 engravings, mailed free upon receipt of four Cents for Postage, to all who mention this book.**

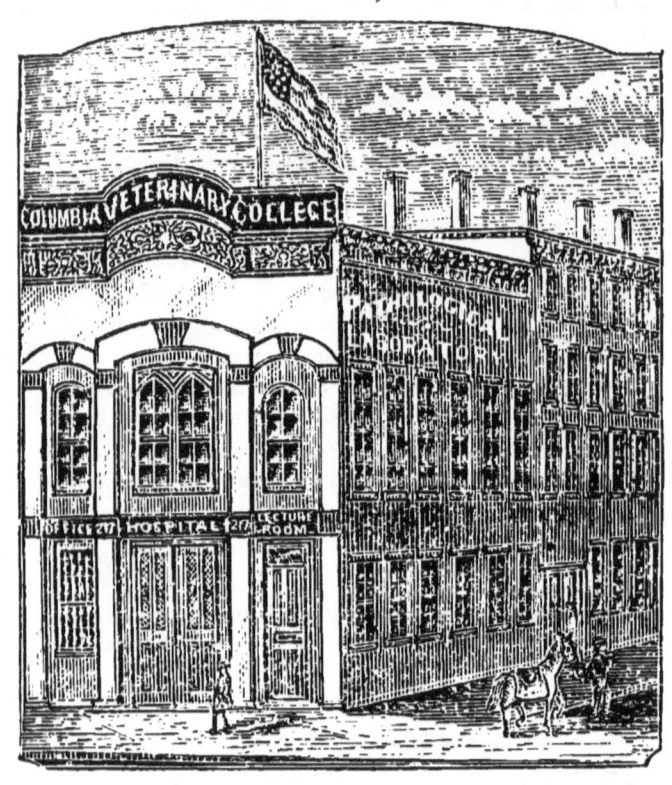

# COLUMBIA VETERINARY COLLEGE

AND

SCHOOL OF COMPARATIVE MEDICINE,

### 221 E. 34th St., N.Y. City.

THE

## REGULAR TERMS OPEN IN OCTOBER.

Has the largest and best corps of Instructors of any Veterinary College in the country. All its graduates in successful practice. For catalogue and further information apply to

E. S. BATES, M. D., V. S., Dean.

# WITHOUT A RIVAL!

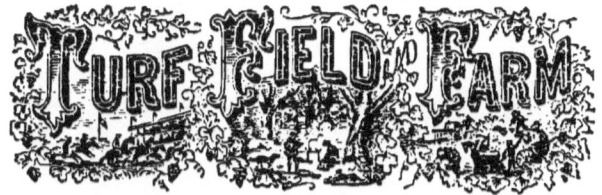

#### OUR STANDARD PUBLICATIONS ON THE HORSE:

American Stud Book (Bruce), 3 Vols............................$25.00
The Horse in the Stable and Field (Stonehenge), 1 Vol.......... 4.00
Racing Rules, 50 Cents; Trotting Rules, 25 Cents.

## TURF, FIELD AND FARM

Has by far the largest circulation of any paper of its class published in the country. Its enterprise, acknowledged ability, independent and gentlemanly tone, have made it the leading Turf Journal of America. As an advocate of elevating and manly sports,

### TURF, FIELD AND FARM

Has won the patronage of the very best and most intelligent people, and the continual increase in circulation all the while is substantial evidence of its growing popularity. The

### TURF, FIELD AND FARM

## IS SOLD BY ALL NEWSDEALERS

### THROUGHOUT THE WORLD.

Specimen Copies, Catalogues of Publications and Premium Lists sent upon application.

Address all orders to

*TURF, FIELD AND FARM,*
39 and 41 PARK ROW, NEW YORK

www.ingramcontent.com/pod-product-compliance
Lightning Source LLC
Chambersburg PA
CBHW030735230426
43667CB00007B/728